Why Are You Mad?

Other works by authors

Genesis
Exodus
Leviticus
Iliad
Odyssey
Hamlet
Tom Sawyer
My Brother Is An Only Child

Why Are You Mad?

The First Significant Advance in Our Understanding of Mental Illness Since We Abandoned Demon Possession

Crawford Harris

Stand Publishers
Nashville

This work is based primarily on firsthand experience, scientific research and analysis. Recommendations contained herein are not to be considered as advice from a medical practitioner.

Harris, Crawford
Why Are You Mad?

International Standard Book Number: 978-0-9794518-1-2 HC
International Standard Book Number: 978-0-9794518-0-5 PB
International Standard Book Number: 978-0-9794518-2-9 EB
Library of Congress Control Number: 2007902051

First Printing: July 2007
09 08 07 8 7 6 5 4 3 2 1

Printed in the United States of America.

Set in Palatino Linotype font.

Stand Publishers may be found on the Web at:
http://www.standpublishers.com

Table of Contents

Dedications

Being deeply loved by someone gives you strength; loving someone deeply gives you courage.

Lao-Tzu

My late, first wife suffered from her own chronic depression, endured living with my manic-depression and brought a great deal of relief, indeed, pleasure and meaning, to my life. Nothing that I am capable of producing is sufficient to honor her as she deserves. It is only with that understanding that I offer this effort to her memory.

My surviving son also bears the burden of chronic depression. I can only hope that this work bears some fruit in helping others better appreciate his problem and, thereby, ease his way.

My daughter is not directly afflicted with a mental illness. Her mother's death, however, placed her in a position, at a tender age, of becoming the source of stability for a family decimated by death and disease. I continue to be amazed at her resources.

Acknowledgments

We cannot hold a torch to light another's path without brightening our own.
Ben Sweetland

It is said with some logic that we are what we eat. It could also be said that we are, in large part, the result of the actions of, and interactions with, many other people. That doesn't roll off the tongue as smoothly as the one related to food nor is the correlation quite as straightforward.

As food is transformed by the digestive system to keep us from resembling a hamburger or french fries, our personality, character and circumstances modify the end result of the interactions of others to something unique. We accept and internalize some of the influences, while twisting others into their opposite or some strange amalgam. The result may not be recognizable in terms of the source but the effect is undeniable. This should satisfy those named herein that they need not accept the blame for any fruit born of their contributions.

My present wife does not understand mental illness but she fully appreciates the difficulty of living with one afflicted by it. She has more faith in me than ofttimes seems warranted. Her support has been necessary.

Dr. Fred Frese identified the particular variety of mental illness I have. Laboring for years under more than one misdiagnosis wasted a great deal of time and limited my ability to deal with the disease. He has also been a friend and an inspiration. Fred is an amazing person. He refuses to let schizophrenia hide or destroy his intellect, his sense of humor, his deep concern for others or his life. His insight, empathy and example have benefitted me, as many others, immeasurably.

Gregory Harris has offered valuable comments on the text and contributed much to my understanding of the roles played by diet and other factors. Discussions with him have helped me develop added directions and nuances to my work with those suffering from these illnesses.

Among those providing various kinds of help and/or encouragement: John Robert Newbrough, Ph.D. of Peabody College, Elliot Valenstein, Ph.D. of the University of Michigan, Linda Campbell, Board Chair of the Vanderbilt Center for Health Services, Robert Whitaker, author of *Mad in America,* formerly of the *Boston Globe,* Brad Wells, Steve Daugherty and Debbie Dykeman.

There are untold numbers of those with whom I have worked in this field who have, knowingly or otherwise, broadened and deepened my understanding and appreciation of the extent and variety of the world of mental illness far beyond my own limited and subjective direct experience.

Foreword

The author, Crawford Harris, consulted with me early in the course of this project. I saw potential in it and offered both advice and encouragement. With this book, I could see the possibility of a contribution similar to that made by Clifford Beers when he published *A Mind That Found Itself* in 1908 (Beers, 1948). Beers described an experience of being three years in a mental hospital. The story generated a wide audience and the support for forming The Connecticut Society for Mental Hygiene in 1912 and, in 1913, The National Committee for Mental Hygiene. The committee evolved into the National Mental Health Association that became a major advocacy group for lay people. Recently it has become Mental Health America.

Mr. Harris describes his experience, like Beers, of living with a severe mental disorder. He has found that the social institutions and the professionals who staff them do not understand the phenomena and do not have effective treatments. In fact, he finds that the treatments are often dangerous and harmful. His mission in this book is to advocate for a different way of conceptualizing the nature of such conditions and for empowering the persons directly affected by them to take some initiatives and to do something about the situation.

His approach is to consider the mentally ill as whole persons who, in their daily rounds, are having problems functioning in various sectors of life. In order to understand them and be helpful, the focus should be on the person in his/her context. Then one looks for ways to optimize the situation so that both the person and the setting are changed for the better. But it has been his consistent experience that the mental health establishment is so committed to an illness model that they can only think of using very specific, usually drug-based, interventions. The Parent-Environment Fit paradigm is of no use to them.

Nicholas Hobbs, of George Peabody College for Teachers, in the late 1950s found himself confronted with a very similar situation. He became aware that children with behavior problems were being diagnosed as mentally disordered and being treated in psychiatric hospitals. Once formally processed, they became permanently marginalized and, after treatment, their behavior problems persisted. His solution was modeled after the fresh-air camp movement (Hobbs, 1982). The behavior problems were defined as learning problems, which could be dealt with best in the context of a special residential school. Prior to referral to the school, children were assessed by a Liaison-Teacher-Counselor (LTC) in the context of the family and a plan developed with the family. Specific goals were set that gave the family continuing responsibility for participating in the re-education of the child. On the weekends, when they returned home, the family was expected to continue the approaches used at the school. During the week, the child worked on his/her plan with counselors and teacher-counselors. The LTC briefed the family as to how the week went and made suggestions as to what the family might work on over the weekend.

This was a program that individualized, that played to the strengths of and was interconnected with the family and the school. This meant that there was both continuity and caring. A two-site pilot program was conducted for several years in Tennessee and North Carolina. At the end of federal funding, it was judged a success and adopted by the Tennessee Department of Mental Health. For several years the new program flourished. But the inexorable pressure of tight money faced the Department. The program was disappeared.

Harris takes an empowerment approach; he advocates the avoidance of the mental health establishment and the encouragement and enablement of persons who experience problems in living. In order to avoid using the generally accepted (and stigmatized) labels of the establishment, he invented two new terms: *Turbiasis* for mental illness and *Agmina* for people afflicted with Turbiasis. As alternatives to traditional treatment, he offers a variety of selp-help suggestions covering diet, supplements, exercise, making friends and using holistic healers. He keeps his emphasis on the current system and does not address the larger issue, how to help the Agmina who badly need treatment. I would urge Mr. Harris to continue his work on articulating his new paradigm and extending it to new policy recommendations.

If one wished to be successful in avoiding the current mental health establishment, it would be necessary to have a workable program and an accompanying statement providing for enabling legislation. This goes beyond the current text.

If I were given that task, I would take this book and *The Re-Education* (Hobbs, 1982) book, and adapt the Re-Ed approach to working with Agmina adults. Then I would take Hobbs, *et al.* (1984) and work on the policy side. Hopefully, Mental Health America could become interested in this project. It could be an effective organization to get such new policy enacted and more holistic programming put into place. If not, Mr. Harris may find a sequel and personal organizing to be effective. Whatever, this book forthrightly places the issue of adequate and appropriate services for the Agmina on the social agenda.

References:

Beers, C.W. (1948) *A Mind That Found Itself* (With a supplement on the mental hygiene movement by C.E.A. Winslow) Garden City, NY: Doubleday.

Hobbs, N. (1982) *The Troubled and Troubling Child*
San Francisco: Jossey-Bass

Hobbs, N., Dokecki, P.R., Hoover-Dempsey, K.V., Moroney, R.M., Shayne, M.W. & Weeks, K.H. (1984)
Strengthening Families San Francisco: Jossey-Bass

Mental Health America's web site may be found at:
http://www.nmha.org/

J.R. Newbrough, Ph.D.
Professor Emeritus
Peabody College of Vanderbilt University
Nashville, Tennessee

Introduction

I write a careless kind of a civil, nonsensical, good humoured Shandean book, which will do all your hearts good -- And all your heads too, -- provided you understand it.
Tristram Shandy (6, xvii)

Only where love and need are one, and the work is play for mortal stakes, is the deed ever really done for Heaven and the future's sakes.
Robert Frost

You are sitting on the edge of a precipice as spectacular as El Capitan. You have a fear of heights. You sit there trying to enjoy the panorama of Yosemite Valley but you are almost constantly drawn to looking down the shear face of this monolith to the base, some 3,000 feet below.

Your mind races. You try to think of other things. You try. You calculate that the height would be comparable to a 300-story building. That certainly doesn't help you think of safer havens, more peaceful or more comforting environs.

You just sit there. You must sit there. You can't leave. For how long? Well, until the bad times return. This is a feeling which is your almost constant companion during those 'normal' periods; the times when you are functional, the times when you are not captive of an episode of depression or some other manifestation of the illness.

Even when your counselor thinks you are doing fine, you live with the dread, the uncertainty, the certainty that if you doze off, if you don't concentrate, if you lose control, you will surely plunge into the depths. Again, this is among the best of times.

The above is not necessarily an experience common to everyone with mental illness. It is not mine now but it has been mine, for years at a time. Others will have different experiences but, as with mine, words will be unable to fully convey those experiences.

This effort, by intent, will combine disparate elements. There is anecdotal biographical information. There are ideas posited which are not accepted as a part of the mainstream. There are descriptions of incidences and attempts to describe emotions that can be understood only firsthand, and only partially even then. There is preaching. There is blasphemy. There is pleading. There are harangues. There is humor. There are opinions. There is education on a vital subject. There is hope. There is despair. But, above all, there is a message, a message that should not be ignored.

We are constantly confronted with new theories and understandings of the nature, structure, chemistry, problems and potentials of the most complex object of our experience. To fully comprehend the brain as the correctly functioning instrument it is supposed to be is likely beyond our capacity. To understand the "broken brain," in the variety of possible manifestations, is surely so.

The limited observations and data, the theories, postulations and mere guesswork that pass for knowledge do have their place, however. They are all we have to work with. They are both the stepping stones and stumbling blocks we encounter along the way.

After 14 years of research, I have fashioned a useful construct from what is available. I have arrived at a place that provides a useful perspective, a valid point of departure. I have attempted to convey my understandings, my precepts, my premises and my inferences to the reader in the hope that we may diminish the dread, the despair, the degradation with which the common misconceptions burden us.

My experience with mental illness may not be unique but I do bring to the table an uncommon perspective. Given, in various capacities, my exposure to a large number of others afflicted with this malady, I also have a broad and deep understanding and appreciation of the more customary experience. I recognize the impossibility of speaking for all my peers but feel that the particular ordeals that have comprised my life, combined with what I have learned from others, make this offering somewhat more useful than a singular, autobiographical sketch.

I see this book as a labor of necessity. It has germinated, almost died and been resuscitated many times. Over this period, I have experienced a range of emotions. These changes are reflected throughout this work. As a reader, it is understandable if the changes seem sometimes jarring, sometimes out of place and sometimes not that readily apparent but it, as my life, to me seems of a piece.

Take a large dose of pedantry, a smidgeon of humility, a well-earned helping of missionary zeal, a less than appropriate serving of outrage, too much egotism and mix unevenly. Spice it with varying degrees of levity, some fitting, some incongruent. The result may be to your taste or it may not. The hope is that it will be but the greater intent is to provide a vital nourishment.

It has been stated that change is the only constant. Without change there will only be what is. That is unacceptable. Two quotes come to mind. The first is from the ubiquitous anonymous. "The more you do of what you've done, the more you'll have of what you've got." If we want a different result, we must change what we are doing. The other is from Bernard Berenson. "Consistency requires you to be as ignorant today as you were a year ago." Would that both you and I can avoid our ignorance of yesteryear.

I have tried to offer sufficient light to allow you to see more, and to see more clearly. I ask that you approach this book with an open mind. If you do, it is my hope that you will see mental illness in a very different light. Reading this book will not make you an expert. In this field there are none. Perhaps, it will cultivate your empathy. Perhaps, it will make you more amenable to accepting new ideas.

In reading this, you will hear different voices. One may be dispassionate, another strident, yet another full of pain, filled with anguish. Several passages are colored by anger, fully justified anger. Immersing oneself in this subject so deeply and for such an extended period is guaranteed to engender a maddening anger.

I have been interested in the subject of the brain, particularly as it relates to mental illness, for the fifty years plus I have had to deal with that disorder. I learned a little, but over those decades an occasional question would present itself. A nagging doubt or two would surface. The answers didn't always satisfy. For one reason or another they didn't ring true but the authorities seemed in general agreement. It was settled.

As I became more involved as an advocate, I felt the need to know more. About 1990 I began an informal, sporadic survey of the literature. Any book or article on the subject that came to my attention was devoured. The more I read, the more frequent and insistent were the questions, the more unavoidable the disparities, the discrepancies and the doubts.

If I could go a bit deeper, it would all make sense. I had to read the research studies. As I began reading these, I quickly realized that it made even less sense. I had to read them critically, analytically. I had to evaluate the study designs, the protocols. I had to reach back and dust off those long-dormant techniques and perspectives of my scientific pursuits. I had to re-analyze these studies.

However rusty I was, it was apparent that much of the literature on the subject was written by and read by people who thought an M.D. degree conferred the knowledge, skills, techniques, temperament and analytical competence of a research scientist. It was equally obvious that they had no clue that they had no clue.

The bulk of the papers available were paid for by the drug industry. The motive for these studies has little to do with science. They have nothing to do with curing mental illness or alleviating the suffering it brings. They are, purely and simply, a means of promulgating the myth in order to sell more of their wares. If a study doesn't support the myth, as the majority fail to do, they keep it from us. Those studies that do support their claims are the result of gross manipulation. Science and scientific method are ignored in their quest for support of their fraudulent claims.

Surely my case is overstated. No. Absolutely not. The Food and Drug Administration accepted only four of the fifteen studies Eli Lilly presented on Prozac. Even those four were the object of severe criticism by the agency. How the FDA accepted them with their noted deficiencies can only be explained by the FDA seeing itself as the defender of the industry, instead of as a legally designated entity created for the sole purpose of protecting the public.

The more I learned of the methods and behavior of the pharmaceutical companies, the more pronounced my nausea. Maybe, if I did a little more research I could convey something beyond the confusion I felt. More research. More concentrated research, and still nothing written but notes.

My predicament was that I was now in the same situation as the real researchers, the neuroscientists. I was well along into being able to tell people what mental illness was not and why it was not, but I still could not tell people what it is.

The leading researchers were making progress. They were making discoveries at an ever-increasing rate. It was just that the pieces of the puzzle didn't fit. Here were more pieces being found but still nothing fit. A question came to me. Did all of these pieces belong in the same box? Were they all parts of the same picture? We had been given the wrong picture.

My investigations had not been limited to what was coming out of the laboratories. Unbelievable stories kept hitting me in the face of the duplicity, the reprehensible behavior of the pharmaceutical companies. Anything they touched was corrupted. The 'chemical imbalance' model was not sustained by the results coming out of independent laboratories. It could not be.

It turned out that the real scientists had known for perhaps four decades that the model was incorrect. They didn't know what caused mental illness. They did know what didn't cause it. And here were the drug manufacturers milking their spurious science with their snake oil nostrums to the tune of multiple billions of dollars each year.

In sifting out the results of studies done by 'researchers' who were not trained research scientists and the results produced from misleadingly designed studies, I found I had eliminated essentially any results sponsored by the manufacturers. I had eliminated any and all studies that supported the illogical and preposterous concept that mental illness is caused by some supposed insufficiency or excess of one or more of only three chemicals in the brain.

My discarding of so many studies from the drug industry is no great loss. The government funds the overwhelming portion all pharmaceutical research despite the image the industry has so successfully implanted in the public mind.

The statements I've made will strike many as unduly strong. Just hang in there. Further along you will find that they are supported by competent researchers, logic and results.

One problem with writing this book was deciding on who was going to be my intended audience. There was no desire on my part to write an academic treatise. I had already seen the level of writing in the journals. While impressing both the authors and the readership, it provided no advantage, if understanding was to be the goal.

I wanted this book to serve a need for the general public. I wanted this book to help begin the re-education of the medical profession and others who serve the mentally ill.

There are, unavoidably, several terms from the medical, chemical, biological and pharmacological fields sprinkled through some of the chapters. I have provided a glossary of the words that might be unfamiliar. Don't feel insulted if I have included words you don't require to be defined.

I asked several people to read parts or all of the manuscript. They represented a wide range of educational backgrounds.

The glossary is there to cover as large a segment of the population as possible. If you come across a word with which you are unfamiliar, go first to the Glossary. It may save you having to pull out your trusty Webster's.

It will be sometime after the middle of the book before you find the end result of my research. The chapters preceding that play an important role in preparing the reader for those results.

My intent was not to develop the outline as a novel, keeping the reader in suspense. My intent was to humanize the subject and to provide you with unfamiliar tools, to plow the field, to plant the seeds for the flowering of new ideas.

You will develop a new perspective, one requiring a different path, heading in an unexplored direction and coming to a somewhat unfamiliar destination. I present a few flowers in full bloom but, beyond that, I offer the neuroscientists several handfuls of seeds and acres of fertile ground.

This is purposely not a scientific paper, disrupted with hundreds of citations. It does offer the researchers a new direction, however. It also offers a task more scientifically rewarding than attempting to turn the sows' ears of the 'chemical imbalance' hoax into silken money bags for the pharmaceutical industry.

Reading the introduction to this point, you might ask, "But what is the book about?" There appear to be too many themes.

Offering nothing more than the description of a new scientific model would not draw the interest of the public I want to reach. If I offer nothing more than criticism of the pharmaceutical/medical complex, people might say that it's been done already. It hasn't been done in this manner.

The theme might be said to be an attack on the priesthood of a secular cult and on the falsehoods they promulgate. These priests are really hucksters. The dogmas they proclaim are a cleverly designed hoax to sell products. The products they offer are essentially no different than the snake oil their itinerant grandfathers sold off the backs of wagons.

The primary difference is that these modern snake oil salesmen are immensely more sophisticated and successful than their forebearers. They make enough money to buy off the local sawbones. They rarely are tarred and feathered and run out of town anymore. They should be but they aren't.

A colleague characterized the present situation regarding mental illness as a crisis. It has been a crisis since the medical profession took over from the Quakers and like-minded people who predominated the operating of sanitariums until the middle of the 19th Century. Since the drug industry and psychiatry convinced the majority of the public that pills were the answer, it has only gotten worse.

The growth in the numbers of people with mental illness and the damage done by the drugs has created a pandemic public health disaster. As bad as the situation is, the public is unaware. They are constantly hearing of new miracle drugs. They are totally in the dark as to the actual state of affairs. They are unaware of the broad social damage and costs that effect everyone.

One can only think that my evaluation is overdrawn if one does not know the reality of mental illness. As a society, we are unaware of the monetary costs, the social costs, the failure of standard methodologies and the inhumane treatment far too many people with the illness suffer.

This book will provide only a very limited look at the problems noted in the previous paragraph. I will provide a short list of books by others who treat those matters more thoroughly than do I.

If you have a mental illness or have a family member or friend so afflicted, you may be interested in learning about the scope of the problem. If you are not in one of those categories, you may have no interest. You may think it is not your problem. Wrong. This is, far and away, the biggest health issue we face.

There is hope. Sadly, not for everyone but there is hope for tens of millions. There is a new direction now available that embodies that hope.

In reality, this book has the same theme as *The Wizard of Oz*. I show you the sham that hides behind the curtain. I apologize for the lack of a musical score and that much more of this is in black and white than in Technicolor but put on your red shoes, click your heels three times and follow me through the lair of the wizards.

I have no Magic Wand and you would hardly mistake me for the Good Witch but I do provide you with a way out of the fantasy land. I give you a map to help you back to the real world; the world of fact, a healthier clime, a more comfortable place that you may call home. Welcome back to Kansas.

The pharmaceutical and medical industries have done the people of this country a great disservice. We spend far more than twice the amount per capita on healthcare of any other country. Yet, our health ranks behind every other industrialized country and several that aren't. Our life expectancy is lower. Our infant mortality is higher.

Side effects from prescription medication are the fourth leading cause of death. Senior citizens eat cat food or skip meals to help themselves afford medication. For the past

20-odd years the drug industry has been the most profitable industry of all. Is this what we want?

This book addresses only the part of the health complex that relates to mental illness. I show the damage that the psychopharmaceuticals do. I show the facts that prove they don't work. I provide the logic that explains why they don't work; why they can't. I relate how the drug companies lie to the public, physicians and the government. I point to the connivance of the Food and Drug Administration and the National Institute of Mental Health in fostering the 'chemical imbalance' fraud.

I provide a new model. It is based on facts and logic. It explains much about mental illness that could not be answered before.

If mental illness and its cause are found to be different, then the treatments need to be changed. I offer a small arsenal of therapies that work.

There will be those readers who, having heard a description of the book, will try to ignore it, having already decided that it is wrong, valueless and written by some benighted psychotic. Too bad.

An essential human quality is the ability to learn. As no rational person claims to know everything, even of a particular, narrowly defined subject, one who refuses to learn has damaged or killed his own human nature. He is no longer a fully functioning human being. Anyone who approaches this predisposed to dismiss it is the truly unfortunate one.

I intend to pull no punches. There is no boss to whom I must answer. I have no professional associations or attachments to influence me to "play nice." I find some support for my approach in the words of James Fenimore Cooper. "Candor is a proof of both a just frame of mind and of a good tone of breeding. It is a quality that belongs equally to the honest man and to the gentleman."

My primary concern is for the well-being of those afflicted with mental illness. Secondarily, my curiosity about the subject is too insistent to permit caving in to those with incompatible agendas. As Bette Davis said in the movie *All About Eve,* "Fasten your seatbelts, it's going to be a bumpy night."

Nashville, January 2007

Chapter 1

Are You Going to China?

We owe almost all our knowledge not to those who have agreed, but to those who have differed.
Charles Caleb Colton, "Lacon"

No man's knowledge here can go beyond his experience.
John Locke

China is a large, fascinating and complex country. To most everyone reading this, China is far away and exotic. They eat different food. They dress differently. They have no alphabet. Few have an automobile. They are rich in history and culture but poor in possessions. They are different.

China is so foreign to our own experience it would be advisable to hire a tour guide. Would you employ a guide who had never been there? You might find someone who has eaten at a few Chinese restaurants. It might be someone whose total familiarity with Chinese art comes from his immersions in the decor of those restaurants.

Perhaps he knows how to say Kung Pao Chicken or Sweet and Sour Pork. He might even have sufficient knowledge of anthropology to know that Chinese people have an epicanthic fold and are generally of shorter stature.

Well, okay. For this trip of a lifetime you decide to engage a Chinese person. But who will you choose? There's more than a billion of 'em. They're all Chinese. Just pick one.

I should warn you. Most Chinese never travel too far from their place of birth. Most may not have a full appreciation of the country's rich heritage of art or history. There may even be a bit of a language problem in some regions. Few will know of appropriate lodgings and accommodations for foreigners. Just being Chinese may be an insufficient criterion for your purposes.

Has your tour guide through mental illness ever been mentally ill? Has he ever experienced the alien nature of rapid-cycling manic-depression? Has he been gripped with the fear of paranoia? Has he heard voices? Has he tried to survive suicidal ideation for months on end? Has he endured the shear terror of losing control? Has he felt the total absence of a sense of self? Has he borne the stigma of mental illness? Has he been to China? Can he help someone benefit from their visit to the fullest? Is he an expert on China?

Has he ever survived that chemical storm in the brain of a schizophrenic? Is he conversant with the internal language of the brain of one with mental illness? Does he have a firsthand familiarity with the interior terrain of the most complex object of our experience?

How many psychiatrists, psychologists or psychiatric social workers have been to China? How many truly know what it's like to be mentally ill? Might they also benefit from a guide?

But what about a person with mental illness? They know what it's like. As you would need an interpreter to speak with most Chinese, most people with mental illness cannot communicate what it is like to those who have not shared the experience.

As with most Chinese, who have never traveled widely in their own country, most people with mental illness are effectively confined to their own experience.

Relatively few people with mental illness have had the benefit of learning about the subject beyond their own experience and what their therapist or counselor has provided. Since those therapists and counselors are unlikely to have firsthand information, most of such interchange would be as useful as the inexperienced foreign visitor educating the Chinaman who hasn't wandered more than a day's walk from his ancestral home. To the extent that such instruction might be of some value, the information flows in the wrong direction.

Faster, faster

I cannot provide you with the firsthand experience. I might impart a hint, a mere suggestion, but it is impossible to offer anything close to conveying the terror, the torment, the frustration, the anger, the confusion, the fear, the emptiness or the desperation that, sometimes separately, sometimes in various combinations, rules major periods of our inner lives.

Imagine running down an incline. Imagine it becoming steeper. You begin to run a bit faster. As it gets steeper, your momentum carries you forward insistently. You feel unable to stop. The angle increases. Now, you can't stop. You have trouble moving your legs quickly enough to keep your feet under you. If you can't move them faster, you will fall.

You know you've reached your limits but the speed increases. You know that you can't keep up. You know you will fall. You know you will come crashing down in a heap. You know you will be hurt. But, at some point during this relentless acceleration, you realize you are experiencing a thrill.

However terrifying the decent, the thrill keeps pace. It can only be likened to a roller coaster on steroids, a roller coaster that twists, turns and contorts but that seems only to head steeply downward. You know you will end up crashing but, strangely, you want the plunge to continue.

The above was an inadequate attempt to create a physical analogy of a manic state I have experienced. I have felt myself, on many occasions, to be in an emotional, intellectual and physical freefall. The uncontrollable, accelerating decent and impending crash were absolutely palpable. They were in no way avoidable.

Accompanying the dread was a feeling that my brain was expanding with commensurate speed. I would lay in a bed strewn with a few dozen reference books. Every question I posed either was swiftly followed by the solution dredged up from some unfathomable depth of my brain or I was able to immediately open the appropriate reference and find the needed formula in seconds. The pace at which my brain expanded increased. The books became unnecessary. My brain seemed to strain only to grow faster, not to comprehend. Comprehension was a given.

I knew that, as with a balloon, there had to be a limit to how much my brain could expand before the inevitable burst. I was scared to an extent beyond experience. I knew that the end, the explosion of my brain, was certain death. But, the growing intellectual power I felt was seductive, awesome. I seemed to be approaching omniscience. Perhaps it was just my personal version of Nirvana. It's difficult to believe that the effects of any hallucinogen could compare.

One might assume the answers that came to me during those episodes were mere gibberish. In fact, two inventions resulted from these episodes. The brain is a continuous wonderment, even when in extreme distress.

Although I cannot provide you with a full experience or understanding of mental illness, I can offer a perspective that is closer to that strange reality than one who has not been there. I can offer a direction that will not strand you on the wrong side of the globe. The percentage of mentally ill who have an understanding of the disease beyond the boundaries of their own personal tribulations is small.

Some of those with that wider grasp may not be capable of articulating their knowledge. They may not have sufficient experience at communicating. They may suffer disabling anxieties. They may not be given the opportunity because the stigma influences providers, family and others to not consider them a credible or valuable resource. They simply may not be inclined to speak of something so personal.

These factors greatly reduce the number of people with mental illness who can, or are permitted the opportunity to, help the 'normals' obtain and develop a more valid, more useful picture, a truer understanding of the subject.

I offer myself as your guide. I speak both languages. I have lived for a considerable time in that place that 'normals' consider alien, exotic and foreign.

As a former executive director of a nonprofit devoted to those with mental illness, I have some appreciation for the problems of others that are not mine. As someone who has counseled others, as someone who has visited in numerous hospitals, institutes, jails, prisons, group homes, private homes and on the streets, I deepened my understanding. As one who was homeless, I can speak to that special situation from experience.

Were these credentials that are particular to one with mental illness not enough, I have had the advantage of other perspectives. I have held elective public office, serving, among other positions, as a commissioner of police. I was involved in developing a program that received national notice for success in rehabilitating prison parolees.

Having been both homeless and a Realtor, I have an understanding of the problems of housing for the mentally ill and potential solutions that is uncommon. My experience in education gives me an insight into those particular problems.

This is not merely a recitation of my background. I have labored long, hard and, to some extent, creatively to find ways of dealing more successfully with the multitude of problems affecting and affected by those various areas.

Even with such an unusual combination of range, variety and depth of experience, I have found myself ofttimes the victim of the stigma of mental illness. Some would ignore the credentials rather than abandon their preconceptions and admit that one with mental illness can enlighten them. It is possible to learn from anyone. To refuse to learn because of a baseless prejudice against the source is both foolish and evidence of unforgivable hubris.

Unexpected lessons

When my eldest daughter was 16 years old, there was a federal Summer program to help children from poor families become involved in the needs of their community and earn some money. She was assigned to a nationally known facility for the mentally retarded. She came home sobbing at the end of that first day. My daughter was brought up in a manner that would be considered old-fashioned and overprotective. That first day she was told to assist a mentally retarded patient with his restroom functions. He was in his early twenties. She was mortified.

I calmed her down. She related the situation. I told her that she needed to return. I told her that she could learn something of value in the most unlikely of circumstances and from anyone, even someone with mental retardation. She was more than reluctant but was finally willing to put some trust in her father's judgment. Within the week, she was coming home excitedly relating her day at the center. She went on with valuable lessons from this. She majored in psychology and made a career in social services to the needy.

Another analogy comes to mind. Were I to present myself as an expert on how it feels to be pregnant and how it feels to give birth, I would make myself ridiculous. At a minimum I should expect snickering. More likely, I would be the object of derision or outright scorn, and rightly so.

Being a male I am not qualified to provide such advice and never will be. It would take more than presumption on my part to even consider playing such a role. It would be totally absurd for me to attempt and even worse should anyone take me seriously. Is it really necessary to point out that 'experts' in mental illness who have no firsthand experience should be met with a similar lack of acceptance of their credibility?

A male physician may explain the mechanics of pregnancy and childbirth but cannot be considered a resource of value concerning how the mother-to-be will experience either. In the case of mental illness, the physician, or other practitioner, has not the knowledge to explain either the experience or the mechanics. Their lack of knowledge and experience seems insufficient reason to keep these people from presenting themselves as experts.

The public's lack of understanding of mental illness allows these people to avoid the well-earned derision and scorn and to position themselves as the high priests of this mystery. While a tour guide to China needs to speak the language, gibberish usually suffices for those who claim to lead us through the landscape of mental illness.

The above may strike some as unduly harsh, or even incorrect. This is just the first chapter. As you will learn later on, regardless of the very successful public relations campaigns of the pharmaceutical companies, no independent neuroscientist in the field of mental illness accepts the 'chemical imbalance' model. The 'chemical imbalance' model is a scientific dead-end and has been known to be a fallacy since at least 1962.

If your friendly neighborhood psychiatrist does buy into that model, he is out of step with those who are far better trained and positioned to know. He has likely paid closer attention to the blandishments of a pharmaceutical salesman and to the monetary benefits provided by the pharmaceutical companies than to the research. Don't follow him to China.

People who buy into the stigma are, beyond the damage they do to the mentally ill, shorting themselves. They are denying themselves knowledge and insights that are unavailable to them from any other source. It is not an indictment of all 'normals' to say they are in thrall to this stigma. It is simply a fact. It also is not their sole preserve.

Those with mental illness also have bought into the stigma. They usually see themselves through that distorting prism. It does its damage to the mentally ill both directly and indirectly. It also afflicts all others.

Is it really that difficult for someone without mental illness to grasp exactly what it is? Even more so. Imagine my likelihood of success in describing various colors to one who has been blind from birth. But that is not the correct analogy. Now try imagining that blind person trying to describe color to someone who is color-blind.

There are others well-qualified for the purpose but, as I happen to be in the vicinity at the moment, please accept my services as your guide. I will not be able to make you an expert but I will be able to offer you a better understanding of mental illness, the people who are afflicted with it and some suggestions for improving our lot.

Turn the pages. Let me introduce you to a world far more alien than China; a world far more immediate than you may have realized; a world far more difficult to translate than calligraphic ideograms; a world far more demanding to navigate than choosing between options from column A or from column B.

Chapter 2

Sticks and Stones

Words may be deeds.
Aesop

I hate false words, and seek with care, difficulty and moroseness, those that fit the thing.
Walter Savage Landor

Whackos. Nutcases. Crazies. Loonies. Mad. The insane. All but the last of these are no longer politically correct. You would be hard-pressed to find a psychiatrist or psychologist who has never used the terms insane and seriously mentally ill interchangeably.

But just what do you call people who suffer from mental illness? Please don't call us mentally ill. You wouldn't refer to someone as a cancer. We are people; we are not a disease. Still, what do you call us?

Over the past few decades the system has gone through several words in its effort to give us a label. Once we were patients. Later we were clients. Now we are consumers.

I thought everyone was a consumer? The term is supposed to indicate someone who is a consumer of mental health services. Here we are being described by what the professionals do for, or to, us - not in terms of our malady or of what we are intrinsically. Perhaps we should consider terming diabetics pincushions or amputees as prosthetic holders.

There was a National Mental Health Consumers Association. It had state and local affiliates. A member of the public once told a board member of a state association that she thought, based on its name, it was an organization devoted to taking people with mental illness shopping. Perhaps the term is just a little too generic.

Some people have been calling themselves survivors; meaning, they have survived the system, not the disease. The problem is that most of this group are the radicals who deny that there is such a thing as mental illness. To them it is all a plot by the professionals to create business for themselves or, more sinisterly, simply to control them.

More would probably use the word survivor to describe themselves as one who has survived mental illness were it not to associate them with the fringe element. Another problem is that groups of people with different issues use the term, e.g., incest survivors, cancer survivors.

One take on the subject is that when you pay someone to perform work for you, that person is your employee or your hired hand. Although we pay the providers of mental health services, directly, with insurance or through government programs, they get upset at being referred to as our employees.

Are they concerned about being referred to with an honorable word which puts them into a subordinate position to people they look down upon? Is this more upsetting to them than some of the denigrating terms they use for us?

A Suggestion

What do you call us? I don't know. Consumer is meaningless and inane. Whatever term is used, it must be something, unlike insane, that carries no negative emotional weight beyond the trauma of the illness itself. You would see someone who physically abused a quadriplegic as despicable. Mental illness plays havoc with the emotions. We have no need for additional, gratuitous assaults to our psyches.

Over the years, the discussions I have heard or been a party to have limited themselves to finding an existing English word that might be appropriate. The present usage of the word consumer is unsatisfactory for any number of reasons. Patient is nonspecific. Client didn't prove acceptable either. Survivor has its own problems. It seems to me that Latin is the most promising avenue to explore.

The medical profession prefers to dignify various maladies and medications with names rooted in Latin. Why not mental illness? Why not those afflicted with mental illness? Terms with Latin roots not only lend some aura of dignity but can help avoid the negative associations that many of the presently used words carry. Once commonly accepted, such terms might help minimize the stigma and the wounding effects of those now in current usage.

I think I have been able to devise a couple of terms that address the above-mentioned problems. The first newly-coined word is Agmina. This would be used to indicate those who suffer from mental illness.

As observed elsewhere in this book, mental illness is rooted primarily in genetics. It is growing as a percentage of the population. It appears to be, at least in part, an evolutionary development. Those who already have this genetic change might be considered to be in the vanguard. The suggested term has its root in the Latin word for multitude and vanguard, *i.e., agmen*.

I would also suggest that it be used as both singular and plural, masculine and feminine. This would conform more to English usage and avoid the problems and confusion we find with a commonly used and misused set of Latin words: alumnus, alumni, alumna, alumnae.

The word vanguard has positive connotations. It is not a word that is likely to acquire negative meanings, in and of itself. Given the numbers affected, there is no denying that we are speaking of a multitude. We are not speaking of the occasional nut or whacko one sees wandering the streets, talking to himself. We are not dealing with the media's caricature. We are contending with a mass which totals, according to what seems the best guesstimate, in excess of twenty percent of the population.

I thought that by changing the root, *agmen,* to Agmina I had created a new word. Later, I found that *agmina* was already a word. Used with the same meaning of multitude, it had some currency in the Middle Ages. It is found most frequently in Gregorian Chants. I doubt that such use will be the cause of undue confusion.

The term mental illness is presently used with a great lack of precision. Many people include any number of mental pathologies and behavioral aberrations. The differences in definition are based on confusion and misinformation and themselves create further confusion.

What this work covers and what is more exactly meant by the term would have been, before my research produced the results it has, more limited and less complete.

Previously, I would have limited my usage essentially to what we currently term chronic depression, manic-depression and schizophrenia. That is how I defined mental illness. That is what might be referred to as the political definition. A better explanation of that and a more accurate and more useful definition is elaborated in a later chapter. First, we need a word to define.

The other word I offer is for the maladies themselves. That word is Turbiasis. Derived from the Latin word *turbatus,* it means angered, exasperated, restless and/or troubled. It is the root of the English word turbulent. Along with a sense of futility, or guilt, or worthlessness, that definition manages to cover a significant part of the emotional spectrum one experiences.

Both personal experience and observation convince me that those feelings encompassed by the Latin word have the most potential for being turned to advantage. Words may be balms or weapons. We need both but we need words that let us say what we need to say.

As the traditional three-headed terminology has proven more apt to be a cause of confusion than a set of precise categories or descriptions, using a single word to identify the various manifestations of a common basic origin seems preferable. By putting the linguistic *troika* out to pasture, we can focus on a more differentiated, more precise and more useful approach to what we are dealing with.

I have only a passing familiarity with Latin. The stylistic variations on the root words, therefore, represent what appeals to my eyes and ears rather than any adherence to the grammatical rules of that language. It might be suggested that some variation on the word proposed for the illness, e.g., turbic or turbistic, could be used to designate those afflicted. The intent of a totally different word for this purpose is to avoid labeling people as a disease.

I have some hope, albeit with minimal expectations, that these words come into general use. Absent that, these lexicographical progeny of mine might lead others to more suitable and/or salable alternatives. In an effort to test their prospects, I will employ them throughout the remainder of this book. I capitalize both. That is my preference as I think it useful to lend every importance to those afflicted by the disease, the confusion and the stigma.

Comments of some of those reading the manuscript expressed one or another problem with my insistence on using these new words exclusively in the following chapters. It seemed imperious, if not arrogant, to impose them on the reader. It admittedly can become annoying or disruptive to the flow of the text until one acclimates to their use. Be assured that there are credible reasons, perhaps misguided, perhaps not.

The terms used for mental illness and its victims have changed frequently in the past. We have had more than one change since Abraham Lincoln was described as suffering from melancholia. If I fail to use these new words here, what expectations can I have that others will accept and use them?

The need for alternatives to presently used terms is explained above. I see the need for change as imperative, if there is to be any success at diminishing the power of the stigma and the confusion permanently attached to our present, unacceptable vocabulary.

The use of these words may seem a bit confusing, at first. I apologize. I have taken great efforts to make this book accessible to the general reader but the nature of the subject imposes certain demands. The brain is exceedingly complex. If we learn something new every day, learning two new words will make this day special.

If some readers feel they have more viable options, their ideas are more than welcome. Perhaps such suggestions may be included in future editions.

Chapter 3

Taking it Personally

How many times I have pondered over my own misery and over death; with what floods of tears I have sought to wash away my stains so that I can scarce speak of it without weeping, yet hitherto all is vain.
Petrarch

Character cannot be developed in ease and quiet. Only through experience of trial and suffering can the soul be strengthened, ambition inspired and success achieved.
Helen Keller

I write this chapter with considerable reluctance and trepidation. It is included with the understanding that it is too narrow in its focus to offer any significant general insight into the subject of Turbiasis. I have been convinced or, more properly, compelled to admit that it may have some value in highlighting what should be obvious, that people with Turbiasis are individuals, that the stereotype is pathetically baseless.

The stigma that haunts us fails to account for that individuality. The stigma is simply another stereotype. As with other stereotypes, it is built on a foundation of misinformation, prejudice and conceit. Stereotypes find a ready audience among the simpleminded and the intellectually lazy. I trust that at the end of this chapter there will be no question that you have met someone who doesn't quite fit the delusional contrivance that is the stereotype.

My intent is to limit this to a very spare sketch, essentially composed of a few factors relating to my own experience with family members who were, or are, also Agmina. The people I have included strike me as having played a role in the development of the personal traits that have contributed to the way I have dealt with my illness. Some have been of help. Others have hindered my progress. Still others have sometimes been a boon, sometimes a hindrance.

The point is that complexity is the hallmark of all people, particularly Agmina. Such a brief, selective portrayal of this complexity hazards this sketch sharing much in common with a poor caricature. Just bear in mind that this is far from a complete picture. I am, as my fellow sufferers, a complex human being, not a disease.

Papa

My maternal grandfather was imposing both physically and in his personality. Only a few inches above six feet, his bearing and demeanor usually translated into a formidable presence. His visage could make the monuments in a town square seem cuddly. He defined the word stern.

I recollect heeding the call of nature while visiting his home when I was likely eight or nine years of age. He entered the bathroom unannounced and saw me holding a strip of toilet paper of perhaps four or five squares. He advised me that anything more than two squares was wasteful, then turned and walked out. The impression he made on me was powerful enough to remain with me to the present, nearly six decades later.

In 1923, he took on three full-time jobs. He became city manager, chief of police and superintendent of the waterworks for a rural county seat. Because of a mandatory age limit, he was required to retire from the position of police chief twenty-two years later but continued to hold the other positions.

He had an atypical form of manic-depression, one which I share. The manic phase is not defined by the more common euphoria, perhaps a feeling that one can fly from the roof or is free of some other human limitations. It is marked instead by a compulsion to do, to accomplish, to overcome some dread of being worthless. Days of sleeping more than three or so hours are rare.

One can experience this manic phase either by itself, concurrently with the depressive state, the depressive phase alone or, on occasion, be temporarily without an active state of illness. As both the mania and the depression can be experienced at the same time and they are not exact opposites, the term bi-polar is inappropriate. It is a form of the malady that seems to match the known manifestations one could see in Theodore Roosevelt.

The picture I sketched above of my grandfather might lead one to conclude that he was some sort of ogre. Perhaps you think that, as a young person, I saw him as just a mean old man. To the contrary, I knew him capable of being one of the most empathic and generous adults of my early experience. He was fortunate to have substantial employment throughout the Great Depression. Given that it was the Depression, in a rural southern town, his remuneration for the three positions he held, although he was more fortunate than many, still left him in a financially marginal state.

One day he saw a man he knew fairly well. Of course he likely knew everyone in that small town relatively well. The man was accompanied by most of his eight children. My grandfather noticed that all were in need of shoes. It just happened to be payday. He and the father gathered the entire brood, marched them down to the shoe store and bought new shoes for every one of the children, over the protestations of the father. I'm assuming that the father's objections were somewhat muted, recalling how I described my grandfather's intimidating bearing.

My grandmother was possibly a full five feet in stature. She was as warm and wonderful as anything Norman Rockwell could conjure. She was also the only human being not afraid to confront this anthropomorphized realization of the immovable object.

When he was unable to produce his paycheck, he was obliged to tell her what had occurred. Her response was withering but couched in her patented sweetness, "You do realize that you also have eight children?"

I was different from the other kids. I was left-handed. The grandfather who so awed, terrified and inspired me was also left-handed. This shared quality drew me to him. With him I was not a freak. Here was a commonality with someone I saw as deserving of respect. He didn't poke fun at me for being different. I wanted him to like me. My grandmother was no problem. Out of her large assortment of grandchildren, I seemed for some unknown reason to hold claim to a special part of her heart. My grandfather was the challenge.

My fondest memories of my time with him also contained just a touch of disappointment. I watched him, with a rapture seen only in little kids, do amazing feats. I was fascinated by his ability to crack his knuckles. This was not just a cracking of knuckles. This was to me the equal of any vaudeville performance. It was an amusement he performed for himself at odd moments. It seemed completely unaffected, not unconscious but almost so. It was somewhat akin to other people humming a favorite tune while stranded in traffic. Perhaps it was merely his method of releasing a bit of stress.

He was surprised when I noticed and flattered when I attempted to imitate him. It turned out to be my passageway to his heart. At first, my little hands were unable to produce any sounds whatever. I was persistent. Certainly, some might use less flattering terms. Okay, yes, I was relentless. I was stubborn. I don't know whether these times were the origin of that particular character trait or simply an example of that now innate feature of my personality. Although I never quite matched his virtuosity, I could show off to my little peers a talent they admired.

Another item in his bag of tricks was his ability to wriggle his ears. I was so proud of myself for mastering this entrancing skill. I could stand in front of a mirror and watch my progress. I could see my technique develop. No longer just a sporadic twitch, I had amplitude, I had control. I was quite accomplished at this exotic skill, I thought.

I wanted to show off for Papa. I performed every minor variation I knew. I was a master, just like him. He then casually showed me his secret weapon. He wriggled one ear at a time. Immediately, I plunged from being a master to nothing more than a tyro.

My disappointment was transmuted into a determination to again join the ranks of the masters. I failed. I failed at that particular expression of the talent but my persistence, or stubbornness, was eventually rewarded. I had the consolation of creating a related trick of my own, one that my grandfather couldn't perform. At the ripe old age of six, I had overcome failure. If not again a master, at least I had passed beyond the novice phase.

Although I subsequently experienced many failures, it might be that this one little success, born primarily of my well-developed stubbornness, provided me with one of the tools with which I fashioned whatever successes I have enjoyed, including the ultimate success, that of surviving.

Stubbornness may be considered something other than a positive personality trait by most but for me is has proven anything but negative. It is rare that any personality trait is truly one-dimensional. The point to keep in mind is that human beings are complex. This is true both in levels that are observable unaided and those at the cellular level.

Yes, I do admit that I find this particular trait hard to tolerate in others. Therefore, I'm not recommending it for you or anyone else, just for me. I have many traits that others would see as less than endearing but the following may offer some clues as to their source.

Mother

One of Papa's daughters was my mother. She was bright and talented. She desperately wanted to pursue her education. She, in fact, earned scholarships to college in art and music. Her father, however, was a man of his time. He was firmly convinced that girls needed no more than an eighth-grade education and felt he had been more than accommodating to allow his daughters to complete high school. He would not be moved by any pleadings she could muster. She saved up her frustrations and took them out on her firstborn: me.

My mother vested all her dreams of expressing those thwarted talents in me. She never realized, or at least never admitted, even to herself, that she was afflicted with chronic depression. Those two factors, combined to make for a less than ideal childhood.

Among the characteristics of my mother's illness, a strong tendency towards obsessive-compulsive behavior was readily apparent, not to a child at the time but to other adults and to me, in retrospect. She set my standard for me. It was simple: perfection. Failure to meet that standard resulted in verbal abuse and/or corporeal punishment. Although not necessarily true in fact, it seemed that punishment was a daily feature of my formative years.

I began piano lessons at the age of four. Later, voice, the clarinet, the organ and saxophone were added. She wanted me to include the violin but was unprepared to purchase a second one for the use of her one left-handed child or to re-string it twice a day.

Required practice was increased to four hours daily for a period. I was constantly reminded that Jose Iturbi practiced eight hours every day. It made no difference to her that he was a professional musician, while I was just a child. While other children were playing games and developing the necessary social skills, I was sitting alone, relating to Mozart, Beethoven, Verdi, Gershwin and several other dead people.

I was enrolled in school early at the insistence of my mother. She had enough of her father in her to get her way with the school authorities. With her tutoring, I was reading and writing prior to entering school. There seemed always to be a great deal of pressure, a great deal of stress. Sometimes, looking back on that childhood, I wonder how I avoided ulcers until my late twenties.

The stress was not from striving to meet the competition, to be ahead of my classmates. That was not a problem. I was considerably beyond my classmates. I never compared myself to others, however. I was programmed to judge myself, and be judged by my mother, in relation to that simple and unwavering standard she had set for me: perfection.

One may presume that I had a well-developed superiority complex. That would not be the case. It was constantly drummed into me that any musical, artistic or academic talents I might have were no more than unearned blessings. One was required to earn them *post facto*. At the time I tended to see them more as curses than blessings. Later, with some modicum of maturity, I came to see them as responsibilities. Advantages were to be shared, not hoarded.

Failure to meet goals or expectations induces stress in anyone. The impossibility of meeting the standard that was set for me guaranteed the feelings of failure. It guaranteed stress. Just as with the stretching of a rubber band, the greater the distance between expectations and actuality, the greater the tension. As perfection was the only standard of which I was aware, it became my own standard.

To be left-handed, to be the youngest in the class, to be the smallest, to be far ahead of my classmates, to miss out on all the playtime, to be socially inept, all of these made me different. Grammar school and, even more so, high school are not especially times when kids want to be seen by their peers as different. One wants to belong. It seems that these are truly the times that try men's souls.

The complex feelings of being different were added to the self-hatred of knowing you were a failure. An "A" on a test was not a cause for pride. It was expected. The teacher bringing attention to some academic effort that she deemed laudable merely highlighted for both me and my classmates my being different. I didn't want my teachers to praise me, to use me as an example. I didn't want my teachers to like me.

There was no challenge in the classroom. When that is the case, the unchallenged child has too much time on his hands, too much time for his mind to wander but sufficient time to disrupt the class. Usually, such a child becomes a discipline problem. So it was with me. Such a situation seems to the child not an opportunity to learn but an enforced, interminable period of inactivity. There is simply too much energy in a grammar school-age child to expect endless quiescence.

Although I was an occasional problem earlier, I recall that it was late in the fifth year of school that I became truly rebellious. That rebelliousness has to be understood in the context of a post-World War II setting. I was not directly challenging my mother and teachers. I was just making no serious effort to study the assignments or use my practice time at music to improve my skills.

I accepted that I was a failure and behaved accordingly. My grade cards became the evidence of failure. Remember, that failure was not in failing grades. I performed well enough to receive passing grades. From that point on, my mother and all of my teachers shared the mantra, "I know you're capable of doing better. You know you are capable of much better."

It may have crossed my mind that there would be a benefit to achieving poor grades. I might become accepted as one of the gang. I recall the pleasure of being somewhat accepted during the first and second grades. Comic books were apparently in short supply due to the war. My dad was a grocery store manager and that worked to provide me with a larger library than the other kids in the neighborhood. Although I was the youngest, we would sit around with me reading to the others. As comic books became more plentiful and they became better readers, my status as being different replaced my temporary acceptance as a peer.

No longer a part of the crowd, I became a target. I was not the first kid ever to be the target of a bully but I think I tried to deal with my situation in a relatively uncommon manner. The bully and a couple of his cohorts would put me on the ground and immobilize me. My chief persecutor would then proceed to tickle me. I assume that I need not describe the feelings of helplessness, *et al*. engendered on these occasions.

I decided to try to inure myself to tickling, to tickle myself until I was sufficiently accustomed to the sensation that it would be bearable. Instead, I discovered something I had not known. One cannot tickle oneself. I adjusted my plan to account for this new insight. I developed the ability to imagine I was trying to tickle myself while being tickled by someone else. I enlisted the aid of my younger brother to practice this.

When my tormentors showed up for their next display of bravery, I simply laid myself down, without their assistance, and spread out my arms and legs fully. They were totally frustrated by my failure to fulfill their need for the perverse pleasure of seeing me writhe and squirm.

I discovered that being different wasn't necessarily being something lesser. I had overcome their brute force with mind, discipline and a refusal to be a victim. It was only a minor epiphany, one of many. It failed to completely alter my concept of myself as inferior but it may have been the first of many steps away from self-loathing.

My father had dreamed of being a professor of history but that dream was dashed by the death of his father when he was a teenager. He retained a love of history and learning in general. It was easy for mother to persuade him to purchase me a set of *Encyclopaedia Britannica* during the fourth grade. It, the shelves of history books, *National Geographic* and an ever growing collection of science books kept me intellectually stimulated and satisfied at home, while in class I was becoming an academic fraud.

My mother's assessment of me as something of a discipline problem and one who needed a more academically challenging setting led to my being enrolled in a military preparatory school. I'm sure her decision had a certain logic to it but it didn't work out quite as she had envisioned. Repeat after me, "stubbornness."

I did not take well to the strict discipline. Another factor was that I felt even more out of place among a group with whom I had little in common. Apparently, being born into wealth bestows an attitude, one that I had no reason nor opportunity to cultivate. I had never felt poor before. Dad made a respectable living as a manager. We were a bit above average in the middle-class neighborhoods in which we lived. Now, with all of my other proofs of being different, I could add being poor.

We moved to a new neighborhood a month before I entered this prep school. Riding the bus and walking home in my uniform let the kids in the new neighborhood know that the new kid was different. I couldn't pretend to be normal and gain their acceptance. While I was seen as the token poor kid at school, when school was out I made the daily transition to being the arrogant little snot in the eyes of the kids in the neighborhood. As with Turbiasis later, the perceptions of others defined me.

At this time, we lived in one-story bungalow. Out front was an unusual plant. It reached a greater height than the house but formed more as a bush than a tree. It had hundreds, thousands of limbs, or shoots, coming from the base. They were probably the diameter of an adult's little finger down to the thickness of a pencil. We called it the bush tree.

My infractions both at school and at home merited punishment. Mother's favorite method involved that bush.

She would break off a shoot and thrash me with it. After breaking one, she would continue with another, then another. She would tell me that she would stop only when I ceased crying. She would lose control.

The blows were not limited to my posterior. The lashes and the marks they left covered from neck to ankles. If I happened to turn my head, I would experience a sharp stinging lash on the side of my face.

The prep school required every boy to go out for a sport each season. They had a swimming pool which we were told covered more than two acres. Everyone was required to go swimming during the warmer months. The lashes usually broke the skin.

The sting of the chlorine was insignificant compared to the stinging humiliation of having to make up excuses for my classmates. I'm certain they found my explanations improbable but it did tax my powers of creativity to develop all of those excuses. The trauma from that was such that I was into my forties before I willingly wore short-sleeved shirts.

After being kicked out of prep school three times in two years, I was back in public school. I saw no evidence that the prep school's reputation for academic excellence was justified. The transitions, in both directions, were not difficult because of any differing academic standards. One of my better behaved schoolmates at prep school was Ted Turner. Yes, that one.

High school was more of the same, with one significant exception. If I was not made to feel different enough already, nature had a surprise in store for me. In a class of over four hundred, I entered the eleventh grade as the second shortest boy. During that nine months, I grew from five feet, two inches to six feet, three inches. I ended that year as the fifth tallest in the class.

Such rapid growth was accompanied by a great deal of awkwardness. The spurt was so fast that it entailed relatively little added weight. Both literally and physically, I was painfully thin. Mother Nature seemed as perverse as my own mother.

Mother, as many with Turbiasis, exhibited somewhat of an unhealthy preoccupation with religion. As it had been up to the point of my graduation from high school, my life was to continue for a while being an attempt to fulfill my mother's thwarted ambitions for herself. Although placing 363rd in my class, I was offered five scholastic scholarships. I was not permitted to accept any of them. My mother had decided that I was to be a missionary. Off I was sent to a religious college.

I intentionally failed all of my religion courses that first year, while doing well in math and other subjects. This eventually persuaded mother to give up on my ever being a missionary and to allow me to enroll in a real university.

That second year I was as a kid in a candy store. History, mathematics, physics, chemistry, biology, astronomy, anthropology, too many choices. My interests were so broad I couldn't decide on a direction, so I took off in all directions.

Many people experience their first psychotic episode in college. Normally, that is a result of the stress of adapting, or rather not adapting, to college life. I was not troubled by that transition, beyond what I just related. After two years of college, I experienced what was then termed a 'nervous breakdown.'

Stress was certainly the precipitant but it was not a stress related directly to college. Rather, I ascribe it to the accumulation of stress, dating back to my early childhood. It came down to the straw that broke the camel's back.

Looking back from several decades, with a somewhat detached perspective and benefitting from an understanding which was totally absent at the time, I find myself amazed at the resilience of that little kid.

Perhaps children are far more resilient than we recognize and have far more resources for dealing with what life hands them than we generally suspect.

The nervous breakdown led to an argument with my parents. The next day I took off for Florida without notice to anyone. That began my period of homelessness.

About 2 or 3 o'clock the first morning of my new adventure I was roused by a policeman. I never really got to sleep. The tiny gnats, sand fleas, or whatever they were, made that impossible. In addition to my eyes, ears and nose, they seemed to find orifices I didn't know existed.

My brief attempt to sleep on the beach leads me to doubt that such is feasible. Since that time, I have experienced considerable back problems. I ascribe them partially to my choice of sleeping accommodations — telephone booths. This period of my homelessness took place during the 1950s, long before it became so popular.

Dropping out of college in the fifties meant your number was going to come up relatively quickly at the local draft board. After a few months of homelessness, I made the unnatural transition to the military.

The structure, the discipline, being told what to do every waking moment was not a new experience for me but it was one that didn't sit well. As much as I detested it, at that particular time, under those circumstances, it was probably a positive in forcing me out of my state.

You might assume that I hated my mother. For an extended period of time that was true. However, during the younger years, the parenting I received was all I had experience of and, therefore, it seemed ordinary. Hate came later, but come it did.

As I became older, it became apparent that there was a difference in how other parents treated their children. My awareness of her Turbiasis was vague at best during those years. Such generalized assessments as 'nervous breakdown' didn't lead to finely nuanced understandings of the problems, their consequences or how to deal with them.

As time passed, I developed a considerable degree of resentment and anger. Maturity finally led to understanding.

Understanding came over an extended period and in no way resulted in a sudden reconciliation. By the time of her death I was able to say and feel that I loved my mother.

There still remained scars. There still remained a distance, not a chasm but enough of a reach to make difficult a full embrace. Warmth was not a prominent feature of my family life while growing up. What developed in the later years was far less phlegmatic but hardly overwhelming in its level of emotion.

Soon Ok

It may be that the English transliteration of my late wife's name was prefigurative, at least for a period. I'm playing a game here with her name. The actual pronunciation of her second name was oak, as the tree.

Falling in love obviously can be therapeutic. Over the years, I came to experience total acceptance. I was accepted for being me, not for the potential I had as the instrument for fulfilling the frustrated ambitions of my mother. Receiving love did not depend on meeting unrealistic standards.

Being the object of unconditional love is not that straightforward an experience for someone unaware that such even existed. I was intellectually aware of its existence. I was aware that it figured in books, in opera, in poetry and in drama. I just had no emotional awareness of it. It was as remote to me as the daily life of a dinosaur. I trusted that there indeed was such a thing but to me it was no more than some alien abstraction.

It took years to realize how fortunate I was. When I met her, I fell deeply in lust. How could I know what love was? I had no consciousness, no understanding of it. To me love had been a word in a foreign language.

My own definition, based solely on personal knowledge, could hardly match what most would intend to convey in their use of the word. It was not a word with unalloyed positive connotations.

It had been employed in my family but the meaning seemed to connote little more than the most basic biological connection, with overtones of obedience.

The 'Peter Principle' states that people are promoted to their level of incompetence. Something of a reverse of that has always seemed to obtain in my personal experience. The greater the amounts and levels of responsibility loaded upon me, the better I seem to function. This has held true in every aspect of my life, whether in familial roles, at work or in other situations.

A spouse trying to adapt to an alien culture, without benefit of appropriate language skills, imposes more responsibility than a normal marriage. Miscegenation brings problems that require developing adaptive behavior. It also requires the building of a stronger bond between the partners, in order to withstand the constant buffeting to which such relationships are subject.

Parenthood brings additional responsibilities that need no elaboration here. Parenting and marriage, even more customary ones, obviously involve stress. As noted elsewhere, stress can be a destructive element in the life of someone with Turbiasis.

For some unfathomed reason, I thrived on these and other, kindred stresses, involving added responsibilities. Similarly, promotions at work or taking on the extraordinary pressures of public, elected offices seemed only to open hitherto unknown abilities and resources. I certainly am not suggesting that such is the common reaction to these particular stresses among people with Turbiasis but neither is it unique. Even among people with Turbiasis, different individuals respond differently to different types of stress.

Not long after I had acquired an understanding of what love truly can be, after years of slowly coming to a full appreciation of love and of my wife, she fell ill. This illness lasted for more than six years. They were years filled with seemingly unbearable pain, years of physical degeneration.

I have, so far, failed to mention a salient consideration. My wife suffered from chronic depression. As it had been for me, our relationship was also for her an extraordinary palliative. In the latter stages of her physical illness, however, her depression came again to rear its ugly head.

Through all of this, I seemingly remained the rock. I was fully functional and dependable. In retrospect it was somewhat as though I were a stretch of pavement, being increasingly undermined by erosion.

Once the weight I bore was great enough and the support sufficiently compromised, as suddenly and completely as the pavement gives way and the sinkhole appears, I snapped. I collapsed. I crumbled.

Devastation. Disintegration. Grief. These words took on a depth of meaning I cannot express.

Indulge me in a slight digression at this point. When a friend loses a spouse or other close family member, never try to console that person by saying, "I understand." You don't. Or, at least they will feel you don't.

If you haven't experienced a similar loss, the words ring hollow. Even if you have endured such a loss, the sentiment doesn't have the effect you intend. The loss is so personal it is seen as quite special, unique.

The bereaved can't imagine that someone else has suffered so great a loss. While, more than thirty years later, I can acknowledge the possibility intellectually, emotionally the scars remain and the old wounds are easily reopened. My advice is to just let them know that you will be there for them.

Denial was absolute throughout those final years. Throughout the pain, the agony she bore, the possibility of death never came to my mind.

There was an instance, shortly after her arrival, that had a profound effect on me. She had arrived in this country ten days prior to the assassination of President Kennedy.

It was understood that she didn't want to leave Korea but her culture told her it was her wifely duty to follow her husband. The assassination held for her a level of meaning that I did not appreciate at the time.

One of her uncles was a politician in Korea. As a young girl, she was at his home with her cousin. They were in a place where, unobserved, they could see her uncle assassinated by two of Syngman Rhee's thugs. The assassination of President Kennedy brought this to the fore.

One would expect her, given her personal experience, to be on the edge of hysteria. She was made of a stronger fiber. Upset, yes, but dealing with it. Additionally, she still was having difficulty coming to terms with the loss of our first child.

Actually, she was only dealing with these superficially. Holding it in was not the best tack. Shortly thereafter her depression hit her full force. I took her to the emergency room. She was admitted. I was made to wait outside. Matters were somewhat under control until they tried to inject her. Her paranoia kicked in and she also kicked. The attendants strapped her to the bed. The commotion demanded my attention. I charged into the room. To see a loved one in such anguish and being stripped of her dignity by faceless factotums, sears one's soul.

I doubt that I politely asked them to remove her bonds but, under the circumstances and, despite my own rising anger, I did not lose all civility and sense. I was escorted out of the room. After some fuming at my inability to help my wife, I sought out the chief resident. I used what little advantage I had available. They had no one available who spoke Korean, save me. I was permitted to return to the room as translator.

After that short period of my absence, my presence and a great deal of reassurance had an adequate calming effect. She was in alien worlds, both geographically and emotionally. As I sat with her, hour after hour, seeing her anguish and torment was intolerable. Beyond being allowed to stay in the room with her, for the convenience of the staff, not the patient, all other requests were denied. The second evening I was able to loose the fetters to release her. We escaped with only a minor confrontation with a nurse who seemed convinced that I was sufficiently angry to jeopardize her well-being. Perhaps a little of my grandfather abides in me.

Parenthetically, my wife retained a not insignificant amount of trepidation, years later, with my involvement in public life. By that time Turbiasis seemingly had been, for both of us, largely overcome and she had developed far more faith in this country's political stability. I did not and would not do it without her support. Despite her concerns, she felt I needed to get involved.

Her ordeal in the hospital is so indelibly etched in my memory and had such emotional impact that even now, over forty years removed, seeing a similar situation portrayed on the screen brings back much of the anger at the frustration, helplessness, indignities and pain needlessly borne by those already suffering from the disease. Seeing it in person, as I often chance to do, is even more difficult to bear. I make it through only because I see each incident as an opportunity for reconfirmation of an obligation to these people and to the memory of my wife.

My Son

Many little boys become closely attached to their mother at a tender age. That wasn't true in my case but it was for my son. It was at that very time that he lost her. Death is not a concept with which a young child can appropriately deal. Such a loss leaves a permanent scar. It also leaves a tremendous hole, an emptiness.

So overwhelming is the loss of a beloved parent at that age, denial is a common way of responding. The children and I were standing next to the coffin for a final goodbye. My son avoided looking at his mother's remains. Instead, he became fixated on the chandeliers hanging from the high ceiling. Given my own grief at that moment, I don't recall exactly but I think he had some questions or comments about the lighting fixtures. Whichever, it was a distraction from the unknowable, the unfathomable.

I was not the most astute observer of others for some period. It did not become obvious to me until he reached junior high school that there was a problem.

His emotional development seemed to have stopped at about the stage he was at upon the death of his mother. His social development appeared to be significantly slower than it should have been.

Despite the emotional and social deficits, intellectually he excelled. By the age of ten he was beating me in chess. Not that I was especially talented at chess but besting adults in chess at that age is not exactly a mark of intellectual deficiencies. The local university sponsored an annual math contest for high school students. Twenty-two schools, both public and private, participated. My son won the contest as a sophomore.

His apparent slow social progress led him to a group in high school that was obsessed with the game of dungeons and dragons. Were it treated as any other game, it would be of little consequence but it becomes for many a lifestyle. That is what it became for my son and his friends.

When video and computer games hit the market, they too were the object of a like obsession. These were kids who felt inadequate to deal with the real world. They sought sanctuary in these simplistic, primitive worlds of fantasy. It's hard for me to understand anyone being content and fulfilled with a world limited by a 21-inch diagonal screen.

My son did progress emotionally and socially, but at a much slower pace than normal. Part of this is attributable to the friends he kept and their chosen *milieu*. Part, however, can be ascribed to Turbiasis. Signs of chronic depression were readily apparent in high school.

This damnable disease had played a major role in screwing up my childhood, devastated my wife, nearly destroyed me and now was threatening my son. It's easy to direct enmity towards a person but how do you focus and express your hatred when the object cannot be personalized? I sometimes felt that I was worthy of the trauma that was my life. But, I could not accept that the others in my life deserved their fates.

Before my wife died, I thought that I was pulling my weight as a parent. It immediately became apparent that she had been doing the heavy lifting. Perhaps a generous person would have credited me with 10% of the parenting. There was no choice. As a freshly-created single parent, I had to transmute into a 100% parent from a very disadvantageous starting point.

I may have had total responsibility as a parent but I did not become a candidate for father of the year. In their maturity my children seem to largely have forgiven my shortcomings during that period.

My intentions were good, as are those of most parents. The intentions did not ensure good parenting though. A 'normal' person raising a 'normal' child well is problematic. Raising one with Turbiasis requires the patience of Job, the wisdom of Solomon and more good fortune than any one person should expect. I had none of those attributes.

The relationship between my son and I became strained. It wasn't because I didn't care. It wasn't because I didn't try. I thought that because I had experienced the illness, because I understood, I could ease his way. It has been relatively easy for me to establish a rapport with many, many others who share this malady. It should have been no problem with my own son. It just didn't work out that way.

My excuse is that a parent is very protective of an ill child. That is fine, to a point. The problem is that the parent easily becomes patronizing and, quite naturally, paternalistic in the most negative sense. We are dealing with a disorder of the emotions; a disorder that normally alters the personality. It is a disorder that is usually chronic and would be perceived as such, even if the prognosis was not. These factors make it quite different than the measles or the mumps.

Knowing the devastation the disease brings and still dealing with the loss of my wife, what might have been a predictable response from another parent might have been exaggerated in me. My son felt smothered and resentful; resentful that, to him, I had taken control with my patronizing, I-know-best approach.

The damage caused to our relationship was done. It took both time and a great deal of work to heal the wounds, but some scar tissue remains. Perhaps a couple of the reasons for the scars still having some residual visibility is my tendency towards excess (since significantly moderated but not eliminated) and his being too much like his old man.

The last few paragraphs present the basis for a less personal, far more general position I take that will upset some people. It illustrates an important point that will be covered in a later chapter.

Chapter 4

Let's Get Something Straight

Never be bullied into silence. Never allow yourself to be made a victim. Accept no one's definition of your life; define yourself.
Harvey Fierstein

Everything should be made as simple as possible, but not simpler.
Albert Einstein

Use the wrong language, and you're dumb and blind.
Salman Rushdie

The primary reason for writing this book is to provide you the benefit of a firsthand experience and an informed understanding of Turbiasis. This effort would be an exercise in futility, however, without some agreement as to the definitions of certain key words and phrases, as I use them.

I am fully aware of the misunderstandings and disagreements attached to much of the terminology associated with this subject. But, whether or not your definitions are consonant with mine, for our mutual purposes it is necessary to know and accept the intended usage within the scope of this book. If you find yourself in disagreement with me, then, upon completion of this book, you may return to the misconceptions previously held.

I do have a need for exactitude in the use of words. Admittedly, I stray on occasion but the trait is deeply embedded. Why I have such a penchant, I do not know. Where it came from is not readily explicable.

Not an explanation, but an example, involves my late wife. Initially, her command of the English language was essentially nonexistent. Over time, she made considerable progress. We at first depended on my linguistic skills, however rudimentary. Later, she took a greater role. I would flip through the bilingual dictionary and mouth the appropriate word when it was not already a part of my limited vocabulary. She later did the flipping.

When she first came to this country, we lived in Los Angeles, a continent away from my family. During a phone call, my mother expressed that she was anxious to meet my wife. A referral to the dictionary was necessary as I wished to translate her sentiments as precisely as possible. My wife became very upset. She wanted to know why my mother feared to meet her. It seems that common American usage of that particular word had not yet made it into the Korean-English dictionaries.

A later incident, after my wife had gained some facility with the language, required her to look up a word. I was then in elective public office and had introduced my wife to our city clerk. The lady was very impressed with my wife. She stated that she thought my wife was terrific.

That last word was the one that brought out the dictionary. She blanched. We hurried away a short distance for a bit of privacy. My wife was perplexed as to why the city clerk found her terrifying.

Even when engaging in normal pleasantries it is still preferable that we use words correctly. I have been guilty of more than one faux pas in each of five languages. They were momentary embarrassments to me but otherwise of little import. The subjects at hand demand a far greater degree of precision than informal social intercourse.

Insanity

This is the big one. Ask every physician you know to define this common word. Ask every attorney you know. Did you, perchance, find some disagreement? Did you encounter some confusion? I guarantee some of your sources will have experienced difficulty in providing you with an understandable, comprehensive definition.

The odds are that not one member of either group will know how to use this word correctly. Why? The members of these professions are trained in their respective disciplines. Insanity is not a legal term. It is not a medical term. Their use, or rather, their misuse of this term follows from their assumption that the word falls within the jurisdiction of their specific academic discipline.

Insanity originated as a political term. The meaning is quite simple and straightforward. Insanity is the inability to function in an acceptable manner in a given society.

Before getting too deeply involved in this particular subject, it may be necessary to clarify a point. The following addresses the formal use of the term insanity. I am fully aware that it is used differently, much more broadly, informally. But, as Blacks would be offended by others using the word nigger while using it freely amongst themselves, Agmina use the term insane, and its variations and alternatives, among themselves but find it offensive when directed at them by others.

If our society considered it acceptable to kill and eat teenage boys, Jeffrey Dahmer would have been sane. Our society does not; he was not.

The system of jurisprudence would, or should, be bound to determine a person sane or insane, as regards a particular act, based upon the determination of society's acceptance, not upon some static principle peculiar to the legal profession. The question of his ability to function in an acceptable manner is another matter.

Psychiatrists have no warrant to confine a person to an asylum if she or he is functioning in a manner within the acceptable norms of the community. The medical profession has no authority to stigmatize a particular behavior as insane unmindful of whether it is acceptable to the society. Despite their professional presumptions, society defines what is acceptable and unacceptable, what is sane and insane.

Although behavior is a concern of the law and occasionally medicine, both professions are dependent upon the society in this matter. If such a decision is a matter for the society or community, it is a political question. The fact that the behaviors we are considering are those of individuals suggests the need to address the matter beyond the scope of the society. The above definition encompasses this need.

There is a criminal court judge with whom I have had a social relationship for more than two decades. A recent discussion with him could only be described as Kafkaesque. The subjects were insanity and Turbiasis. Reasonably well-educated, at least in the forms and minutiae of his profession, he could not grasp the simplest concepts of the subjects at hand.

Having been a full-fledged member of that dubious fraternity, I have firsthand knowledge that hubris is endemic among our public servants. But it was with a weird combination of amusement and distress that I listened to the unappreciated confusion which is the basis for his judgments on these matters.

Even after another attempt to delineate the differences between insanity and Turbiasis in the most elemental fashion, I was faced with the statement that, "Anyone who commits a crime is mentally ill." I regret not asking him why he didn't find every criminal coming before his bench 'not guilty by reason of insanity.'

If everyone shares the same classification, that classification essentially loses all meaning. It is difficult to fathom how someone can admit of ignorance on these topics while maintaining such strongly held convictions about them. Of even more concern is when that person is in a position to control others, using his ignorance as the basis for his decisions.

I watched an interview on television related to the Washington, D.C. snipers. The interviewee was either a psychiatrist or a psychologist, a profiler, purportedly an expert on serial killers. One statement from this supposed expert floored me. In discussing a particular case, he said that it was obvious that the person was not an Agmina. Why? Because there was evidence that the crimes were planned.

While it's true that people with Turbiasis might commonly be in a state that is disassociated from reality, with their ability to plan being impaired or nonexistent, to say that the presence of planning is proof that the person is not an Agmina is evidence of the 'expert's' ignorance, not of his untutored conclusion.

Maybe I gave him too much credit. It might have been that he didn't consider an Agmina intelligent enough to formulate a plan. If the 'experts' are so in thrall to the stigma, how much can we expect of laymen? Perhaps he was unaware that Winston Churchill was an Agmina or that he played some small role in the planning of World War II.

Insanity is not merely functioning in an unacceptable manner. It is the inability to function in an acceptable manner. If a man is caught robbing a bank, our inclination is to assume that he made the decision while aware of the option not to rob the bank and was capable of following that option. If our assumption is correct, he is not insane; he is considered just a bad person.

The act may have been acceptable to him. Perhaps, that it was unacceptable to society meant less to him than his own judgment. The possibility of capture and punishment were insufficient deterrents. His judgment may have been bad. He may have been stupid. He may not fear punishment. He may not have expected to be caught. He may have been coerced.

Since we have assumed the ability to act differently, he is not considered insane.

Robbing a bank is a serious act, often with serious consequences to the felon and/or others. If the cause were insanity, although just as serious, it would be another matter. In any case, however, it would be a serious act.

While on the criminal aspect of this subject, there is a matter that strikes me as somewhat confusing. Admittedly, I have not delved into this to any great extent but press coverage sometimes brings it to mind. With some regularity, I hear the phrase, "competent to stand trial." In the situations to which it relates, there is the consideration of the defendant's sanity.

We have had the recent spectacle of the trial of a woman accused of killing her five children. As with most spectacles, we are treated to more scintillation than substance. We had the perfect example of lawyers and legislators presuming to know what they were doing.

The law they crafted is the result of their confusion and ignorance. They reached back to the Britain of 1843 to include, and then to misapply, a standard meant for entirely different circumstances.

They blithely stand on a formulation that predates modern psychiatry. This standard pertains to a defendant being able to 'know' right from wrong. It has a place but is inappropriate and irrelevant to the subject of insanity.

The standard may properly be used to decide whether a child has reached a level of maturity to be able to distinguish right from wrong or fantasy from reality. It may also be needed to assess whether a person with Down's Syndrome or Alzheimer's has the capability to appreciate the differences between right and wrong. The standard has its place. It's merely that that place is not in a law delineating insanity.

Why is it digressive? I defined insanity above and, referencing that definition, I fail to find any mention of an awareness, understanding or appreciation of right or wrong. Such a standard is not included as part of the definition of insanity because it has no place there.

As to the question of right and wrong, there are complexities when dealing with Turbiasis. During a psychotic episode, there are possibly factors which skew any reckoning of right and wrong. There may be a voice that one identifies as authoritative telling one to behave in some particular manner or to commit some specific act. In various individuals, that authority could seem to be a god, the president, an agent of some clandestine government agency or some similar figure. There might seem to be a rationale that trumps normal behavioral codes. The act may appear, or the authority may confide, that it is necessary to save the nation from its enemies or the person, or their loved ones, from eternal damnation.

Did Saint Francis of Assisi know right from wrong? We named a city, San Francisco, after a man who ran through the streets of his home town completely naked and screaming. He was trying to get away from the voice of God.

Another factor to be considered is paranoia. This is common among Agmina, to a less dramatic extent, even when not experiencing a full-blown psychotic episode. Would you ask someone suffering from extreme paranoia to refrain from self-protection? One should be able to see that a perceived but delusory need for self-defense can disorient a person sufficiently to make a judgment of right and wrong differ from one made under more normal conditions.

Every sane person makes allowances for their standards of right and wrong to change. Every sane person accepts the fact that right and wrong can be situational. Were it not for such situational ethics, it would be difficult for a nation to find people willing to defend it. Were it not for situational ethics, the sale of handguns would not be a thriving business.

Thou shalt not kill is hardly treated as universally applicable or as an eternal constant, even by the most devout defenders of the faith. We find in the Bible that God resorted to situational ethics on those occasions when he commanded that certain people or groups of people be killed. King Saul was denied the honor of having the Messiah come from his lineage because he failed to obey a divine order to kill. He was punished for not killing. If sane people are permitted to indulge in situational ethics and God sets an example in that vein, why are Agmina to be held to a different, more stringent standard?

Sane people can justify and are permitted, sometimes commanded, to kill under certain circumstances. It should not be difficult, therefore, to comprehend that people who know right from wrong but are experiencing a psychotic episode might see themselves as being in a situation that commands behavior that they might otherwise see as wrong.

Recall that insanity is a political term. Its boundaries are set by the society. Society may presume to determine right from wrong but, in a judicial setting, this question is not suitable for such simplification.

Using the McNaughton Standard of 1843 to determine whether a person appreciates right from wrong, is to place the ball in the defendant's court. It becomes, not society's standards, but the defendant's understanding of right and wrong. To use it as a criterion for sanity, means that the jury has to determine and use the defendant's mind-set at the time of the commission of the crime. That would seem an exercise fraught with insurmountable difficulties, absent a Ouija board.

Insanity is insanity. It need not be elaborated upon, particularly by those ignorant of what it is. There is no need to strictly hold those who are insane to a standard which the sane are allowed to alter as they see fit.

It is only proper that the defendant should be competent to assist his attorney in his defense. I have no problem with delaying the trial in such instances until sanity can be assured. It seems, though, that sanity at the time of the criminal act usually is what evokes the question of competency at trial. Those are entirely different matters.

Insanity is commonly episodic. The phrase 'temporary insanity' is not, therefore, especially helpful and certainly is not descriptive of a rare state, as the media and the legal system routinely seem to suggest. One could be insane at the time of the criminal act but not at trial. The reverse could also obtain. Obviously, either sanity or insanity could be in play at both times.

As one's state need not be the same at both times, sanity at trial should not determine the validity of a claim of insanity at the time of the act. There does, however, seem to be a prejudice among jurors, encouraged by prosecutors, to deny the claim of insanity at the time of the act, if the defendant appears competent at trial. The term 'temporary insanity' has become a pejorative, comparable to 'taking the Fifth.'

Let us now consider an act that is, to our society, of somewhat less moment.

We would be hard-pressed to find someone who has never wanted to just roll over in the morning instead of getting up. We do not normally think of staying in bed as proof of being either bad or insane. We do not expect the courts or physicians to become involved. If we do not go to work, we may lose some income or even our job but society at-large does not find it to be too serious an act; it certainly is not considered a crime. Is it insane, however?

There have been several periods in my past when the depressive phase of my manic-depression was so overwhelming as to make it impossible to leave my bed. Other than for quick trips to the bathroom and the refrigerator, I would remain in bed for two or three weeks. Was I lazy? To those without an understanding of the nature and power of Turbiasis, and initially including myself, the answer was obviously yes. Just get up. Snap out of it.

As disruptive as it was to my life and that of my children, it was not a crime. It was not of major consequence to society, or even my physician. Was I lazy? No. Was I insane? Yes. Even if I had not had the responsibility as a widower of raising two young children alone, society would not have considered my behavior acceptable. My employer didn't. My parents didn't. My friends didn't. Children and Family Services would not have approved, had they known, but, as the children were unharmed, it did not constitute a crime.

Was I insane? My behavior was unacceptable. I had no ability to force myself to behave acceptably. Just get up? Would that be a reasonable demand of someone just out of heart surgery?

The disease eventually progressed, or abated, to the point where I was capable of behaving acceptably, *i.e.*, getting out of bed. Was I insane? Yes. Was I dangerous? No. Am I usually insane? No. Is Turbiasis insanity? It may play a role in bringing about some episodes of insanity but, no, it is itself not insanity.

A person may have Turbiasis and be sane or insane. A person may be 'normal' as opposed to having Turbiasis, and be sane or insane. Insanity, whether in one diagnosed with Turbiasis or one otherwise without psychiatric problems, is usually episodic. It may be a single episode or it may recur with varying degrees of frequency and severity. Turbiasis and insanity are not interchangeable terms. Agmina and dangerous are not synonymous. Even insane and dangerous have different meanings.

If you were not aware of the definitions and of their differences, don't fret. At the time of the hearings on the sanity of Jeffrey Dahmer there was a national television interview show discussing this matter. The participants included two nationally-known psychologists and a professor of psychiatry from Columbia Medical School. During the entire hour all three used the term "seriously mentally ill" interchangeably with the word insane.

Their misuse of the terms did not lead to any confusion on the part of the audience; it merely reinforced the audience's misunderstanding. If those claiming expertise and holding positions of dominance in the system are so lacking in the most basic understanding of the words upon which their profession is based, we suffer as much from the system and its high priests as from the disease.

Misuse of the word insanity should stigmatize the user as confused or ignorant of the subject. It is probably advisable merely to ignore anyone using the words insanity and Turbiasis interchangeably, particularly those presenting themselves as ordained and pedigreed experts on the subjects.

Turbiasis

It would seem advisable, in seeking a definition for this term, to consult an expert. This usually is understood to be a professional in the field. As mentioned above, the professionals are as free and inaccurate in their usage of the terminology as one would expect from any member of the general public. If this appears as an indictment of the professions, it will become apparent that it was earned.

I am tempted at this point to comment that the person afflicted with Turbiasis is the expert. This is not necessarily so. Whatever the illness, the patient normally relies upon the professional for an explanation. With Turbiasis it requires comparing what the professionals have to say with one's own experience, along with a considerable amount of research and analysis. Perhaps a better option would be to ignore the professionals, look to your own experience and study the subject.

First, we must make a distinction between Turbiasis and mental health. Across this country we find mental health centers, mental health institutes, mental health associations, mental health professionals, etc. There seems to be an avoidance among these groups of identifying themselves specifically with Turbiasis.

This may be unfair. Which came first, the chicken or the egg? Is it merely a result of the lack of precision with which they use the terminology? Is it that Turbiasis alone does not provide sufficient revenues?

It could be that writing this has made me more aware of what is being said with regard to what Turbiasis actually is. It could be that there are more opportunities to give the subject play as cable and other media need to slake their tremendous appetites for something to fill all of that air time and column-inches. It appears that knowledge, understanding and expertise are not among the criteria employed by the media any more than it is with those professionals claiming expertise on the subject.

A recent interview of a medical researcher elicited a curious statement about "Alzheimer's disease and the other mental illnesses." Despite his confusion, Alzheimer's does not fall within the scope of Turbiasis. A series of shows on "mental illness" covers depression, manic-depression, schizophrenia and attention deficit disorder - just those four, nothing more, nothing less.

There is a company which has been advertising heavily for some time. The commercials and late-night infomercials speak of curing anxiety and depression. They offered a free audio tape.

I called the phone number and was assaulted by a very sophisticated hard sell. It was relentless. Initially, the combination of "anxiety and depression" just about gave to me the impression the two were of the nature of Siamese twins. As the barrage progressed, however, it became simply "anxiety."

As he finally took a breath, I was able to squeeze in a question. I asked if their program was directed more toward anxiety than depression, as that now appeared to be the emphasis. My customer service representative was quick and facile. His immediate response was, "Oh, anxiety is the cause of depression." Sure, and pain is the cause of tooth decay.

The rah-rah, inspirational hucksterism may work for the occasional person dealing with a relatively mild case of situational depression or anxieties which are not too deep-seated, but the confusion their 'service' presents and fosters is a great disservice to anyone with a case of Turbiasis, a serious situational depression or acute anxiety. Anxiety may be a standalone malady but it can be a symptom of depression or other forms of Turbiasis. To aver that anxiety is the cause of depression is a sign of ignorance, not exactly a qualification for curing a complex, devastating illness.

I have even heard a few Agmina claim that anxiety always accompanies depressive episodes. That may have been those people's experience. Indeed, it may even be relatively common but it is not a universal experience. While I have had many depressive and manic episodes during the fifty or so years I have demonstrably been afflicted with the illness, I have had no more than three or four incidences of anxiety attacks. None of them lasted more than an hour. None of them were associated with major depressive events. While inconvenient and discomfiting, none of them were close to being totally disabling. Whether or not there is any connection is problematical but all of them occurred while I was on tricyclic medications.

Anxiety does not cause depression. It is not necessarily a constant companion of depression. Anxiety, however closely associated with depression, does not qualify as a cause.

It is disconcerting to be put into the position of having to cut through the clutter of all such confused 'expertise.' It is disconcerting to realize that such charlatanism is accepted as expertise by both the general public and those suffering from Turbiasis.

Have you ever tried to wrap your arms around the trunk of a full-grown Sequoia? Turbiasis alone is a sufficiently complex subject to defy mastery. To throw a number of other subjects in with it and claim expertise over the entire array is a bit disingenuous.

Turbiasis is a subset of the spectrum of problems coming under the rubric of mental health. In the past I have most commonly restricted my use of the term Turbiasis to chronic depression, manic-depression, dysthymia, cyclothymia and schizophrenia. For those who are unfamiliar with dysthymia and cyclothymia, they are milder versions of chronic depression and manic depression, respectively. Being the ones I am most familiar with, I continue to use it frequently in that restrictive sense, even though it is broader than that.

Many of the numbers and percentages to which I refer, and are commonly used and widely quoted, are based on that delineation. It's not practical to have a nonprofit or a cause dedicated to fighting disease, all diseases. To be effective there must be focus. Efforts must be constrained to an identifiable, defined area. Those working in the field have therefore narrowed the scope of their efforts to the big three. As these efforts are aimed primarily at government, society, communities and such, I refer to depression, manic-depression and schizophrenia as composing the political definition of Turbiasis.

Anxiety can be one of a number of common symptoms of Turbiasis. Severe, standalone anxiety also qualifies as its own separate illness, as will be shown later. An explanation of the criteria is implicit in the description and definition of Turbiasis to be found in its own chapter.

Mental health includes Turbiasis, along with such other matters as: marital difficulties, addictions of various species, personality disorders, problem children and living with problem children, anxiety, dysfunctional family relationships, sociopathy and even living with a family member who suffers from Turbiasis. This list are not necessarily exhaustive; it simply indicates the many disparate problems that can be confused with Turbiasis when people, especially the putative experts, are sloppy in their use of terminology or ignorant of the differences.

The impossibility of mastering the subject of Turbiasis alone puts into question whether anyone can seriously claim expertise on it, much less on the range of problems classified under mental health. Being a psychiatrist, psychologist or a social worker working in the field of marriage counseling, grief counseling, addictions or a similar area does not qualify one as an expert in Turbiasis. In dealing with the most complex and least understood of all illnesses we need qualified specialists, not part-timers. Turbiasis is a grave malady.

One of every six people burdened with Turbiasis attempts suicide. It would be considered unethical and unconscionable for a dentist, or even a podiatrist, to treat a brain tumor. It is no more acceptable for a marriage counselor to treat Turbiasis. It is a common occurrence, however.

It should be emphasized that situational depression, although not considered by many to be as serious as the chronic versions, can be extremely serious. Just as with chronic depression, it can be overwhelming and destructive. It likewise ofttimes results in suicide. It is impossible to differentiate between the two based solely on symptoms. Although they appear similar, except in duration and cause, they have been perceived as different. As you will see, there definitely is a commonality in the etiology. Situational depression usually persists for perhaps six weeks to six months, even without treatment but its seriousness argues for close monitoring and, possibly, one or more of the treatments recommended in a subsequent chapter.

Providers

The word provider is, as with others current in this area, somewhat unsatisfactory, however charmingly generic. As most commonly defined, it refers to those who provide services to the Agmina.

Many think of this term restrictively. They use it only to apply to psychiatrists, psychologists, social workers, mental health centers, mental health institutes and such other people, groups and facilities dedicated specifically to the subject. Given the needs and necessary interactions of Agmina in a wide variety of situations, a much less restrictive definition is required. There is no need to elaborate on reasons for inclusion of those listed above. We will just concentrate on those who are providers but usually not cast as such.

The closing of more than ninety percent of the beds in the institutes since the nineteen-sixties has saved the states tremendous sums. Those savings are only apparent if one does not look beyond that one budget item, however.

The jails and prisons house many more people with Turbiasis than do the remaining mental health institutes. That they house us is undeniable. That they provide other services is problematic.

The horror stories coming out of prisons and jails, that relate to the treatment of Agmina, are countless. This is in no way an indictment of all the personnel of these facilities. It is, rather, an imputation of the system. Although the prison systems are badly lacking in this regard, the fault is better, if not more profitably, laid at the feet of all of the legislatures and governors.

One should not expect those trained only to control a population of inmates to be expert in their dealings with manifestations of Turbiasis. Wardens, guards and other employees of these prisons and jails commonly are given little or no training or resources for properly dealing with and relating to this special population they find in their care. When training is available it is universally improper and inappropriate. The general conditions of imprisonment, the requirements of security and the social conditions that develop in prisons and jails do not lend themselves to ideal treatment regimens or optimal opportunities for improvement.

Where there is an attempt to provide qualified personnel, the mistakes are to be expected. Taking the advice of the experts, they hire mental health personnel. These people must try to cover the entire range of issues which that implies. Substance abuse is major problem among the population of prisons and quite naturally receives a strong emphasis. This is fine but fails to address all of the concerns of our focus. However significant and obvious the problems related to substance abuse, Turbiasis affects an estimated thirty to thirty-five percent of those imprisoned. We will later discuss important commonalities and connections between substance abuse and the classic forms of Turbiasis.

Many of those providing mental health services in the prisons have no background in the field at all. Since prisons do not receive payment for their services from insurance companies, *et al.*, they are not required to abide by the rules of those organizations. Unless the state legislature imposes some requirement that the personnel be licensed and credentialed, prisons can and do hire a hodgepodge of people with an assortment of unrelated experience.

As poorly as credentialed social workers are paid, not having to employ them allows for paying even less. Actually, this lack of need for credentialed workers could be a blessing, if it were taken advantage of properly. Those duly licensed and credentialed have been indoctrinated in the ignorance of the profession. Proper training would find more fertile ground among the uninitiated. They offer a *tabula rasa.*

I acknowledge that there have been some efforts, scattered, spasmodic and fitful, to train prison personnel but those efforts are totally inadequate and almost wholly misguided. Whether they recognize or admit that they fall under the heading of providers of service to Agmina and whether they actually provide any services beyond housing and misguided therapies, they are a very important component of this group. They are providers.

And then there are educators. They find themselves in essentially the same position as wardens and prison guards. Providing services to people with Turbiasis is not their primary focus, nor is it something for which they have been trained. A teacher's motivations for being in that field may be quite different than the motivations of a prison guard for being in his chosen career but both are forced to confront situations for which they are unprepared. Again, a lack of intent to be a provider and a lack of suitable training does not exempt them from being a member of the community of providers.

As with the members of the groups already mentioned, family practitioners often find themselves confronted with Agmina and their problems. What little they may have covered on this subject in medical school was insufficient to prepare them for properly diagnosing and dealing with the problems they confront.

While they and physicians in other specialties often are the recipients of 'education' in this area by the pharmaceutical companies, the result is not a competency in treating Agmina. The result is both potential and actual tragedy.

A person suffering from Turbiasis very well may not be aware of his need for specialized help or may be reluctant to seek appropriate help. Family practitioners should be trained to recognize the disease and be aware of it, regardless of the malady for which the patient presented himself.

It is also necessary for these physicians to understand the delicacy which is often required in broaching the subject with the patient. Family practitioners do have resources available to them in the form of seminars and such but these commonly are provided by psychiatrists or other family practitioners who presume an expertise that is not necessarily genuine.

The pharmaceutical giants simply add to these problems. Their marketing to physicians and their advertising to the public pressures general practitioners to become little more than drug pushers to the Agmina and those who might be merely hypochondriacs. The success of the drug companies in becoming the dominant educators of physicians is seen in the fact that non-psychiatrists write approximately eighty percent of the prescriptions for psychopharmaceuticals.

Often the front line of this battle takes place in hospital emergency rooms. With psychiatric institutes commonly requiring certification by a physician before admittance, police, who see a case of Turbiasis that requires no special training to diagnose, are forced to lay the burden at the doorstep of an emergency room. Sadly, although a physician may have the requisite credentials to officially sign the certification papers, s/he is no better qualified to deal with the problem than the policeman. Here is simply a required additional burden laid upon the staffs of already overtaxed emergency rooms.

The police play a critical role in numberless instances. They don't always acquit themselves well. Again, this is another case of the system being much more to blame than the man on the beat.

If thirty-five or forty percent of homeless are Agmina, there is no way for the police to avoid involvement. They are also called to homes by families to deal with situations fraught with complexity. How departments can justify not properly training their forces is difficult to understand. What training is available is essentially worse than worthless. It is harmful.

Courts are employed, among other reasons, to make determinations of involuntary commitments. People suspected of Turbiasis cannot be confined unwillingly in most jurisdictions beyond a specified number of days. Three is a common limit. This can be extended for weekends, holidays and any other excuse for the convenience of the judges, psychiatrists, attorneys . . . everyone's convenience, save that of the patient.

I have yet to meet, or even hear of, a judge properly qualified to render judgment on the subject. Some judges require expert testimony to aid in making the decision. That indicates an intent to make an appropriate decision but that simply puts the court in the position of making an untutored judgment of the qualifications of someone else.

Many lawyers will have clients who are Agmina. It may be for a confinement hearing, a criminal complaint, child custody or any number and variety of other issues. Sanity may be in question. Each client, whether with Turbiasis or not, is entitled to competent representation. Ignorance on the subject does not translate into competence. Retaining a psychiatrist is not the same as having an expert witness or resource.

One might expect a difference of opinions in an adversarial situation. Sometimes differences are appropriate, sometimes not. The answer to two plus two shouldn't elicit too much controversy. Death by the stab of a sharp instrument or a gunshot is likewise amenable to general acceptance. Some areas are fairly straightforward. Psychiatry is not one of them.

Psychiatry has not reached the level of maturity that we acknowledge in other disciplines. Psychiatric testimony is never 'expert.' Psychiatric testimony is opinion. It is usually either opinion based on ignorance or on financial considerations.

Lawyers and judges are forced into the role of provider. It has been rare, however, to find any of either who have actually and intentionally provided anything to the advantage or best interests of Agmina.

Once again, we run into a situation of overworked, untrained or improperly trained providers with inadequate resources. The jailors, the police, the educators, the legal profession, the family practitioners and the personnel of emergency rooms all have this unwanted problem imposing itself upon them. None are properly prepared or given adequate resources. But, they are providers.

Elected officials also fall into the category of providers. The problem is that they fail to act as such. Not too many budget items have more appeal to politicians as targets for cuts than those related to Turbiasis. Agmina are heavily represented in the lowest economic strata. Our message is easily ignored by legislators whose sole *raison d'etre* is reelection.

When multiplied by the immense number of those afflicted with Turbiasis, even the ten cents *per capita* expended on research of the subject is a sizable expenditure. Providing services is far more expensive. Spending large sums on the politically voiceless just doesn't have the appeal of a tax cut or a 200 million dollar playpen for professional athletes.

Not only am I an Agmina but I am also a family member of other Agmina. One of my grandfathers bore the burden of manic-depression. My late wife and mother suffered from chronic depression. A son, a sibling, a nephew and a sister-in-law are likewise afflicted. Family members also fall into the category of providers.

Being a family member is far from easy. I touched, in Chapter 3, on the difficulties I had as the father to a son with chronic depression. I also warned you that my experience lead me to a position that would upset some people. Buckle your seatbelt.

The National Alliance for the Mentally Ill undoubtedly has the highest profile, the greatest name recognition, of any organization dealing with the subject of Turbiasis. They are wont to call themselves the 'Voice of the Mentally Ill.' I call them presumptuous. Whatever they call themselves, they are, first and foremost, an organization of family members of people with Turbiasis.

I obviously meet the qualifications for membership. I have been invited to and have attended their national conferences. I have attended the meetings of some of their state and local affiliates. I have participated in meetings with government agencies to which they were parties.

I must have missed the appropriate meeting at one of their national conventions but remember being told that I, and the others in our group, had been made honorary members. I don't say this to brag. I don't consider it anything of which to be proud. This is merely to show that I am familiar with their organization.

One positive aspect of my familiarity with NAMI was finding that the problems I had with my son were not unique. Neither were the causes. The paternalism and patronization were apparently almost universal. The love and concern that engendered these were also common to the members of the organization.

So, if the members of this group have love and concern for their family members with Turbiasis, what possibly could be wrong with that? Let me count the ways. The patronization and paternalism of the individual, that I earlier described in my own situation, becomes the operational attitude of the organization. They see themselves as the authentic voice, not just for family members but, for and of the Agmina.

They see themselves as capable of articulating and defending the needs and rights of their children. They see their family members as incapable of articulating their own agenda. They, as much as any group, have bought into the stereotype, the stigma. This is ironic as they pride themselves on putting forth a great deal of effort attacking the stigma, however misguided and unsuccessful.

Since they see themselves as the 'voice' in the vanguard shouting against the stigma, they cannot conceive that they are victims of it. Their poor little kids need their help. Their kid may be 40 years of age by now but to them he or she is still a child. I understand perfectly. The motives of the members are not in question. Their attitudes towards their loved ones and their actions are. By the way, if my math skills are not too deficient, their five-year plan to eliminate the stigma is a bit overdue.

While the motives of the individual members are not in question, the same cannot be said for some of the leadership and staff. Any large organization is in danger of taking on a life of its own, quite apart from the original impetus. Almost all organizations succumb. NAMI is not an exception in this regard. The organization wants to grow, larger and more powerful. Its goals, its standards must prevail. In this case, they must prevail even against the wishes and interests of the ones they presume to serve.

You find that difficult to believe? When you are trying as an Agmina to advocate on behalf of your peers for a point or position on which the group agrees and find NAMI and/or some of its affiliates fighting you rather than supporting you, it is not difficult to believe. It is difficult to believe the first few times, at least. It soon becomes apparent that the consulting they do with you, if any, is just perfunctory.

They are going to push their own agenda. They will compromise with the government agency or other entity, to enhance their influence. They are willing to wheel and deal when required, but not with Agmina.

They have resorted to *ad hominem* arguments, both at individuals and at Agmina as a whole (primarily the suggestion is that we are not competent to formulate realistic positions). It is a question whether it is more galling to have it done in your presence or behind your back. They have plenty of practice at both.

As an Agmina it is not unusual to lay the blame on yourself. It must be me. Maybe I and my peers are wrong. Maybe we deserve to be treated as less than competent, less than full-fledged human beings.

Given the advantage of meeting with others across the country, you find that they have experienced the same. Maybe we're not as these voices of the mentally ill portray us. Maybe we are entitled to our own points of view. Maybe, just maybe, we can speak for ourselves.

My intentions were unimpeachable in my dealings with my own son. That alone did not assure that my efforts were either in his best interests or fully appreciated. Father doesn't always know best. The lessons I learned from my personal experience, eventually benefitted my son and me.

Experience is the best teacher but learning from someone else's experience is considerably cheaper. Rather than get angry at me for sharing a crucial lesson, learned firsthand, I hope that some members of NAMI and others with loved ones in the same situation will profit, will start repairing the damage done by the natural inclinations of parents.

If you are one of the few not yet offended overmuch by a perspective that hasn't been highly advertised, you will read later on about the horrific hoax known as the 'chemical imbalance' theory.

It appears that the 'Voice of the Mentally Ill' has, for a number of years, been owned by the pharmaceutical industry.

Can this be more than the rant of some disgruntled miscreant? How could he make such an accusation? Surely there's no substance to such a farfetched claim.

NAMI began receiving around four million dollars a year from the pharmaceutical industry in 1996. That is about four million dollars a year more than they have received from the Agmina. I suspect that drug makers see NAMI as their own personal mouthpiece, not as the 'Voice of the Mentally Ill.' I don't suspect, I know that they get something of value for their largesse.

Even if such a questionable financial intimacy did not appear to pervert the professed goals of the organization, their failure to provide an effective disclosure taints them. NAMI doesn't just accept these alms with appropriate gratitude, they do so with unexpected enthusiasm.

While the Food and Drug Administration imposes a few restrictions on how far the pharmaceutical manufacturers may go, how extravagant their claims may be, an organization such as NAMI is unencumbered by the results of studies. NAMI takes full advantage of this freedom.

In speaking of atypicals, longtime executive director Laurie Flynn proclaimed, "These new drugs truly are a breakthrough. They mean we should finally be able to keep people out of the hospital, and it means that the long-term disability of schizophrenia can come to an end."

I have found no glut of people formerly disabled by schizophrenia hitting the job market. There are more leaving the hospitals but most are sleeping on the streets or end up in our jails and prisons. I find no qualifiers in her statement. No "Maybe." No "We hope." No "Possible." I find just flat out flackery.

A review of fifty-two studies of atypicals at Oxford found no advantages of either efficacy or reduced side-effects. Such difficult decisions. Who do you believe, independent researchers at Oxford University or someone bought and paid for by the drug cartel?

It is not hard to find advertising, sponsored by NAMI and smaller organizations, that makes claims that the drug companies are not permitted to make. While the claims are easy to find, I have yet to find a disclaimer, an admission of the relationship.

Despite the false claims, these ads are most helpful. They clarify on whose behalf NAMI and the other groups advocate. Whatever the original intent of its founders, however pure the motives of the bulk of its membership, NAMI has become a front for the drug industry; nothing more, nothing less.

I sometimes need a break from my research and writing. Usually, I plop down and push my recliner back in front of the television, just trying to clear my head and reduce the stress with something mindless. If I have sufficient energy, I scroll through the channels for the news (I said I wanted something mindless). Sometimes something else will catch my attention.

A few months back I ran across a movie that was unfamiliar to me. I don't recall the title. It was likely a recycled made-for-tv movie. The subject was schizophrenia. It actually was more of a love story that revolved around schizophrenia.

The girl who was afflicted was treated poorly by her family. They were not generous and accepting of their daughter. Her fiancé was. He stuck by her. In the end she triumphed. It was clear that the point was that love and support play vital roles in dealing successfully with this illness.

It was a surprise, therefore, to see the final scene followed by a black screen with a message in white letters. The message was to the effect that schizophrenia is a serious disease and one should see a physician to get a prescription because drugs would help.

This screen was followed by another. It suggested getting more information by contacting NAMI. I probably should check it out to see if my suspicions are correct that the movie was funded, in whole or in part by the drug manufacturers.

At a minimum the pharmaceutical industry and NAMI cooperated in the presentation of that film.

Oh, is that all they do to purchase the 'Voice of the Mentally Ill?' No. They have loaned at least one top executive to NAMI to help them improve their operation. They have paid legislators from Texas, where the laws are more to their liking, to speak in other states at events sponsored by state affiliates of NAMI.

There are lots of other such questionable aspects to this liaison but it would be too depressing for both the reader and me to continue in this vein. The relationship is incestuous and unlikely intended to ensure that the efforts of either party place the interests of the Agmina foremost.

There is a person who I knew well for a number of years. His house was only three to four miles from mine and I have been there often. He served as president of a state affiliate of NAMI. He served as a member of the national board and as President of NAMI.

I am unfamiliar with what or how much he received as president but I do recall his bragging when he was on the board about the new luxury automobile a pharmaceutical company provided him for his personal use. He was also proud of the stipend they provided.

I do not know, but deeply suspect, that the same or some other drug manufacturers contributed heavily to his several unsuccessful campaigns for public office. Most towns seem to have one of these perpetual candidates who is never deterred by an embarrassing lack of support at the polls. Our town had two.

When there was an issue between an organization of Agmina and the state department of mental health concerning the latter's malfeasance, misfeasance and nonfeasance, this very active member of NAMI volunteered to go on television to criticize the Agmina and render total support to the state agency. When the state agency refused to respond to three rapes of patients in one of its psychiatric hospitals, there was one of NAMI's most active members standing side by side with the state, against the victims.

Many people, many groups of people provide services to Agmina. Some intend to serve us. Some do not. Some intend to serve us well. Some do not. None are appropriately trained. None, beyond the pharmaceutical and medical industries, are adequately funded.

With so many people involved, one might expect that the overall effect would be positive. Even allowing that many intend to improve the lives of Agmina, I cannot judge any group of any type of provider to have given us an overall positive result. Intentions alone have proven grossly inadequate.

Even the addition of reasonable levels of funding would have minimal or no positive impact. We need the intentions. We need a vast increase in funding. But, without a change in direction and ridding ourselves of the rapacity of the drug companies and the compliant collaboration of the medical community, significant improvement in the lot of Agmina is foreclosed.

If every class of provider is doing more harm than good, we have added the burden of the system to the burden of the disease. Turbiasis is unique in the field of medicine in this regard.

This assessment is admittedly bleak. It is bleak but rooted in the reality of my own experience and that of a host of others. Is their reason for hope? I don't know but I have no other rational choice than to forbear and acquit myself as though there is.

Depression

Character One: I'm depressed. I'm overweight. I don't like my nose. The weather is dreary. I don't like my job. I was passed over for a promotion. I have too many bills. My team lost. My car broke down. My flight was delayed. I'm really depressed.

Character Two: I've been diagnosed as having chronic depression. I'm depressed.

Two people say they are depressed. There must be some commonality. There is. It might be compared to one person having a sprained ankle, while the other has had his entire leg amputated, perhaps both legs. They share the experience of difficulty in walking.

The subject is chronic depression, a disease. The subject is not sadness nor unhappiness, nor normal mood changes. Very few people respond to dreary weather or their team losing by committing suicide.

It is relatively easy to distinguish manic-depression and schizophrenia as separate and distinct illnesses. Chronic depression, however, is frequently confused with situational depression, grief, sadness, disappointment and similar adverse moods.

There are people with chronic depression covering a wide range of degrees of severity. There are people with situational depression covering a wide range of degrees of severity. Some people will experience situational depression to an extent which is totally incapacitating for a period of time. There are those with chronic depression who will not become totally incapacitated. The differences may not be obvious or apparent.

At one time, significant economic downturns were called panics. The powers that be thought that a milder word would be helpful. They hit on the word crisis. That still seemed too evocative of a state less pleasant than what the powers that be wanted conveyed. Well, they thought, let's find a milder word, one less scary. Their efforts gave us the relatively mild word, depression. The search for even less disturbing words has now given us recession, stagnation, stagflation, downturn and a softness in the economy.

I say this to make the point that the word, depression, fails to elicit a full appreciation of the devastation that is supposedly described by its use. Perhaps we would be better served to work our way backward through the list of words used for financial downturns. Although inadequate, crisis and panic come much closer to evoking the emotional state than depression possibly could.

Mentally Ill

I know that I failed above to fully convey the immense difference between depression, on the one hand, as normals commonly use the word and as they think it defines the disease and, on the other hand, the devastation that clinical depression is, or can be. The following may similarly fall short.

In the part above on insanity I mentioned the judge cavalierly stating that anyone who committed a crime was mentally ill. As bad as that stupidity is, more people than I care to think about have gone even further. It happens with such frequency I have come to expect that every time someone finds out about my involvement as an advocate, writer or educator on the subject I will hear the sentence, "Everyone is mentally ill," or, "Well, everyone is at least a little mentally ill." It is like fingernails on a blackboard.

To so grossly misapprehend Turbiasis is to ignore the real, the immense and intense suffering, the trauma of millions of people. To so grossly misunderstand Turbiasis is to demean us, to debase and minimize our anguish and all of our torment.

It may not be the most ignorant or most upsetting, most disconcerting or most offensive statement one could make but it is in the running. Those making that observation should kick themselves in the ass or punch themselves in the mouth a few hundred times.

So, what is the definition of mental illness? Should we go to the medical profession? Maybe the psychiatrists know. Not really. There is not even a single physical marker for any psychiatric disorder.

There being no biological tests for the various mental illnesses, psychiatrists are free to classify what they want as an illness. They may classify these as vaguely and broadly as they choose. To think they do not is to ignore the changing fads as depicted in the different editions of the Diagnostic and Statistical Manual of Mental Disorders.

When definitions of these illnesses change with no changes in the theory and no pertinent new scientific information, the reason is either fashion, politics or money. Psychiatry has taken advantage of this situation to triple the number of labeled mental disorders in the latest version of the DSM compared to its predecessors. I await the next version with every expectation that there will be additions and that the pharmaceutical companies will find that existing drugs, or their clones, are efficacious for these newly-minted maladies.

The drug and psychiatric industries will provide us with definitions that make them more money. Labeling something as a disease or disorder without any understanding of its causes is unscientific, foolish, a waste of time, misleading and a diversion from potentially useful efforts. Rather than rely on the money changers at the temple for definitions, we will address these more specifically and precisely further on.

There are other words that need to be defined for most readers but I felt that the ones in this chapter needed some explanation, some elaboration and some context. Some of the others are defined in the Glossary in Appendix II.

Chapter 5

Is the Earth Flat?

As far as the laws of mathematics refer to reality, they are not certain; and as far as they are certain, they do not refer to reality.
Albert Einstein

In theory, there is no difference between theory and practice. But, in practice, there is.
Jan L.A. van de Snepscheut

Is light composed of photons? Or is it waves? It appears to be both. In dealing with various aspects of light it is only possible to treat it as particles. At other times it is explainable only in terms of waves. To our minds this presents a paradox. Perhaps it is a factor of the peculiarities of our language. Perhaps there is another explanation. Whether real or merely perceived, paradoxes do exist.

Is Earth flat? It depends. Certainly we have proof that it is round. Everyone has seen the pictures taken from space. There was sufficient proof even before the recent advent of extraterrestrial vehicles. How can there be any doubt? Again, it depends. If you wish to take an airplane across the Atlantic, you would hope that the pilot takes the curvature of the planet into consideration. The National Aeronautics and

Space Administration would have difficulty in placing a satellite in orbit around a flat world. The Earth is round.

The Earth is also flat. Farming today has not changed from the Fifteenth Century because of the voyages of Christopher Columbus. To the farmers of old, the world was flat. So it is today. It would need to be a fairly large house for the architect and contractor to factor in the curvature of the Earth. The surface is curved. So what? Most people go through their daily routine without complicating matters by taking into consideration the actual shape of the planet. Are they wrong? Not really.

What has all this to do with Turbiasis? The brain is a far more complex entity than light. Our understanding of both is incomplete but we have had sufficient understanding of light to turn it to our purposes in previously unimagined ways. Even without an accurate perception of the shape of the planet, people were quite successful in accomplishing the varied tasks necessary to daily life.

The primitive state of development in our understanding of the brain should discourage anyone from thinking that the latest explanation is the final one. We would not have suggested that a pre-Columbian farmer not work his fields until the matter of shape of the Earth was settled. We should not criticize his error of ignorance if his perception was functional and useful to his purposes.

Unless we use the limited knowledge available to us in our quest for understanding, we will make no progress. A complete explanation will not appear out of the blue. We are obligated to use that which is available to us, if it is functional and utile.

All of the foregoing is simply to say that I am aware of the possibility, indeed the probability, of being proven incorrect in my explanation of the nature of Turbiasis but it is an explanation that has proven sufficiently correct and useful to my purposes. I have no intention of using it as the basis for neurosurgery or chemical experimentation on my peers.

A significant difficulty in dealing with complex issues is often language. Some problems with our use of language are due to errors in conceptualization. This appears to be the case, on various levels, in dealing with Turbiasis.

Divide and Conquer

In the medical model this is similar to the problem once afflicting the subject of cancer. As long as cancer was seen as 'The Big C,' there was negligible progress in both understanding and treatment. Although cancer is cancer is cancer, it was not until the medical research community began the process of differentiation that progress was made. There may be a hundred different types of cancer.

We now know that whereas all cancers are to some extent describable in a basic set of attributes, there are significant differences in various types of cancer. It appears there is no 'Silver Bullet.' We have found effective treatments for some forms of leukemia which are totally ineffective for other forms of cancer. Differentiation is the necessary perception that some diseases, regardless of family similarities, must be seen more discretely. When lumped together their differences are minimized. Important information is lost.

The medical community chose, at a point in the past, on the basis of both limited understanding and misunderstanding, to linguistically divide Turbiasis into three parts, *i.e.*, chronic depression, manic-depression and schizophrenia. This division was artificial, as it was not in concert with reality. It was insufficient to delineate and describe meaningful differences. Most importantly, it retarded the understanding necessary to make progress.

In the real world psychiatrists and psychologists have been forced to recognize the inadequacy and limitations of only three possible diagnoses. So we find agglutinative terms, such as manic-depressive-schizo-affective with paranoia and anything else the practitioner can come up with to cover the problems she or he finds.

They wind up in the dead-end of some terminological tangle. The imprecision also accounts for the fact that most people diagnosed with Turbiasis for more than a short period of time have received more than one psychiatric label. This causes confusion for everyone, most particularly the patient. The result is often a natural distrust of the profession. This distrust is usually seen by the professionals as further evidence of the Turbiasis or evidence of further mental problems or personality disorders.

The professional providers in this field are wont to see themselves as laboring in a science-based field. They are not. Even if they were it would make no difference, as they have not been trained as scientists. There are studies showing better results by shamans, witch doctors, than by the professionals who dominate the field in advanced countries. Perhaps, once they have attained the level of shamans, they then may aspire to credible science.

The state of the art at present is woeful. It is confused and based on assumptions that have no basis in fact, defy logic and cause untold misery. Such a description hardly suggests a scientific endeavor.

The reader may resist and protest such a characterization. It may be premature for me to depict the situation so, to draw such an unflattering picture of the present system and its practitioners. I will begin soon to elaborate the foundations on which I base these assertions. If you hold a conventional view, you may be surprised, shocked or offended by the opinions stated above. That is good. That is necessary. I am not rearranging the deck chairs on the Titanic.

The basic postulations of this field are wrong. They are harmful. They impede progress. They use resources that should be better employed. They bring misery and forestall hope. If the present theory is wrong then it is likely the associated therapies are wrong and, therefore, useless or harmful. If we change the paradigm, we must develop new therapies and treatment strategies.

The results of my research suggest a treatment strategy and a few specific therapies. If, as I show, this new paradigm is useful, others may use it as a point of departure to develop additional therapies and, in due time, perhaps even an assortment of pharmacological agents.

As I will explain further on, Turbiasis is Turbiasis is Turbiasis. We encounter the same problem with Turbiasis as we did with cancer. In a sense, all Turbiasis is fundamentally the same, in the same fashion as all cancer is fundamentally the same. But, inside a particular category, such as depression, we may ultimately find fifty differing types. And so, there may be fifty different forms of manic depression and as many varieties of schizophrenia.

I spoke in terms of these three categories but the diversity that in fact exists across the spectrum eliminates the need and the usefulness of the present categories. We may even add other illnesses to this unholy trinity. To ignore or to be unaware of this diversity is unacceptable. Attempting to treat this variety of illnesses with the limited, inappropriate arsenal now being used is foolish. The comfortable, profitable little world of psychiatry is about to experience a change of terrain underfoot on a scale comparable to that of the world of mariners at the end of the 15th Century.

Agmina and all others experience Turbiasis far differently. The perspectives of the former have been ignored. This is not helpful. A great deal of value and potential in these perspectives have been lost in the attempt to understand and deal with the problem that is Turbiasis. This is an attempt to redress the absence of these viewpoints.

No claim is made that what is presented herein is all there is or is sufficient to balance the scales. Some of it will seem harsh to those who are encumbered and constrained, willingly or knowingly, by the prevalent orthodoxy. For those who feel attacked by this alien *Weltanschauung*, it might be profitable to remember that much of what they do and have done, much of how they approach the subject is not merely alien to Agmina; it is and has been insulting, degrading and painful, even to the point of death.

Much of the orthodoxy fails to ring true to Agmina. It sounds distorted and phony to those who have firsthand experience. It has, however, become so dominant, so pervasive, that the majority of those assailed and assaulted by it have accepted it. It is not unusual for Agmina to doubt and distrust their own experience. It is the norm.

Being able to find Agmina who buy into the 'chemical imbalance' marketing strategy is neither difficult nor validation of its credibility. It fails every test. Finding victims who accept the untutored claims of those whom they embrace as authority figures may be proof of other things, but not of scientific merit.

What is Turbiasis? What is its nature? What is common to all of its forms? Many people, professionals especially, have spoken the word cure in connection with Turbiasis. Until we have brain transplants, there is no cure. That may not strike you as the hope you were looking for or expecting. It isn't but just hang in there.

Structure

Turbiasis has to do with the structure of the brain. Its structure is not, under normal circumstances, susceptible to any change which might be considered to represent a cure. We may cut some of it out, We may disrupt connections, as in a lobotomy but that does not change the structure of what remains.

We may disrupt or kill a few billion cells through electrical shock but that does not repair the basic structure. We may inundate it with various pharmacological agents but that does not change the basic structure. Short of a change of its structure, there is no cure.

It is probably easiest to describe the brain of someone with Turbiasis with an analogy to transistors. Back in the days of electronic tubes we had radios, television and even computers. The advent of solid state electronics brought several advantages. Lower costs, reduced heat and smaller size were among the advantages. There were some disadvantages. A prominent one was the inability to generate the huge wattage needed by broadcast stations. Ofttimes, when nature provides us an advantage, it compensates with a disadvantage.

The brain of one with Turbiasis can be likened to a transistorized or solid state computer. The brain is significantly more densely packed than is normal. There are more neurotransmitters, more neuroreceptors, more synapses, more dendrites, more axons. This, in a sense, means the brain of one with Turbiasis is potentially more efficient or has greater capacity. More brainpower is compacted into the same sized space. Nature makes us pay a price, however.

With more neurotransmitters we have more chemicals coursing through a stimulated brain than is normal. As long as the neuroreceptors can keep up with the flow of chemicals through the brain, not only does it function acceptably, it often functions, in some respects, in a manner superior to what is considered to be normal for a brain.

Imagine you had identical twin ladies sitting next to each other, one afflicted with Turbiasis, the other not. This may be genetically less likely than with normal twins but let's accept the premise for the sake of illustration. If you told them they were both beautiful or told them they were both ugly, you would get reactions from each of them. There would be a difference between the two, however. The brain of the one with Turbiasis would have a greater chemical flow than the other. She would have a heightened response neurologically and possibly otherwise as well.

So you have more chemicals coursing through the brain than normal. So what? If there are a sufficient number of neuroreceptors in proper working order, the brain functions adequately. If not, you have problems.

One aspect of this may be, to a point, appreciated by normals. Perhaps you have been in a dangerous situation. Let us say you are driving along, then a person or another vehicle darts out into your path. You know you are in danger. You know to put on the brakes, swerve or both. But you are momentarily frozen. You can't react. The problem is a rush of adrenaline. It temporarily overwhelms the capacity of neuroreceptors and other elements of the brain.

It doesn't mean you are incapable of thinking. It doesn't mean you are incapable of properly assessing the situation. It simply paralyzes you for a short period of time. As frightening, and perhaps dangerous, as such an experience might be, the feelings of helplessness are short-lived. Can you extrapolate? Can you imagine such a state enduring for weeks, for months, for years?

Beyond the feelings experienced for a limited period, the persistence of those emotions incurs a range of other problems and questions. Is this permanent? Am I different? Why am I different? Different means not as good as normal. Am I less worthy? I am less worthy. I deserve to be this way. This just highlights some of the process and progress of feelings one goes through with Turbiasis. In an attempt to explain it, it is necessary to use words. But words cannot convey the reality, the terror, the anguish, the trauma.

How the above and similar questions are answered determines both one's self-image and behavior. It brings changes in one's personality, not just episodically but usually on a permanent basis. Hence, we commonly find personality disorders that must be addressed.

There is commonly another problem associated with this compactness. With significantly more potential connections in the brain, we often experience a couple of results. One is a decrease in speed and/or efficiency.

If many more elements of the brain are available in a particular process, *e.g.*, memory, calculation, analysis, it should not be surprising that the brain sometimes involves more elements, makes more connections, in a given process than a normal brain might. Making these extra connections requires more time.

People with Turbiasis often, in varying degrees, require more time to complete these common functions of the brain. Do you translate slowness as a sign of lower intelligence? You shouldn't. It takes longer to digest *War and Peace* than the associated Cliff Notes.

The preceding paragraph may give the impression that this slowness is present in every Agmina, or consistently present in some or all. That is not the case. The brain is too complex for such easy generalizations and facile conclusions. It is too complex to allow such a simple explanation to be comprehensive.

An increase in density can mean shorter connections. We find that Agmina will, in some circumstances, sometimes exhibit greater speed in various functions of the brain.

It is said that anything simple enough to be put on a bumper sticker is untrue. The necessary elaboration of political opinions and other such thoughts which a car owner deems worthy of our notice are too complex to be given ample explication by the simple assertions allowable within the constraints of a bumper sticker. One shouldn't expect any simple statements on this subject to cover all of the possible contingencies.

More connections means more complexity, which opens the process to more opportunities for breakdowns. By this, I am not referring to so-called emotional or nervous breakdowns.

The normal brain experiences an occasional lapse of memory, miscalculation, *etc.* I simply mean that, as with a more complex machine, a more complex brain is more susceptible to those same phenomena. The more parts and connections, the greater the opportunity for mishaps and glitches.

The second potential result of this complexity can represent an advantage, a disadvantage or both. The longer route, with necessarily more connections, means that there is more opportunity for making connections which lead in other, unintended directions.

Tangential thinking appears to be significantly more common among many with Turbiasis. These tangential forays may lead to dead ends. They may also lead to interesting or useful ideas or perceptions. This would be termed creative thinking.

Using the same recipe for every meal, one will seldom experience a different taste. Consistently thinking in the same patterns is unlikely to lead one to anything new.

DNA changes frequently. The results of such changes may not be significant, or even noticeable. Most such changes are not. Some result in changes that are beneficial to the organism. The majority, however, result in changes that are not beneficial. Many, in fact, may be harmful.

The changes are not driven by some overriding pattern intended to promote progress. The changes are essentially random. That is one reason why Charles Darwin used the term 'natural selection.' Those which are harmful generally find no future.

Ideas and perceptions, in much the same way, have the potential to be significant or not. They may be positive, negative or neutral. The majority of creative, *i.e.* out of the ordinary, ideas will likely be of no value. Only a precious few will be worth pursuing. The difficult part is actually evaluating the results to determine which ones might have value.

When you hear someone saying things that seem crazy or weird to you, you may be right. The person may just be having a creative moment, one without appropriate evaluation. Then again, you may not be properly attuned to recognize or appreciate the latest incarnation of the hula hoop or see the potential for societal and cultural change represented by the next technological miracle; the television (invented by an Agmina), the personal computer or the Internet.

There are Agmina living in their own special reality, completely unrelated to the real world. There are also Agmina who are in the process of shaping your coming reality. Sometimes it is not that easy to match each with their true role.

Did you find this description of Turbiasis satisfying? Did it answer some questions and address some of the aspects of the behavior, capabilities, limitations of those afflicted with the disease? Did it seem too simplistic? Did it conflict with what you thought you knew about Turbiasis? Did you find the holes? Did you realize that it is provably incorrect?

Wrong

Some years back, the early 1960s, there were autopsies of the brains of Agmina taking neuroleptics that found a greater than normal number of dopamine receptors. There have also been other autopsies showing differences in the morphology of the brain in Agmina.

This lead some to the conclusion that there was an increased density, an increased capacity involved in Turbiasis. That does not appear necessarily to be the case but it does provide us with another way of looking at the brain.

Despite the fact that the above model can successfully account for several aspects of Turbiasis, it is, as I explained, provably incorrect. It may, however, be of some help as the 'Flat Earth' model has its place.

What I find odd is that the 'chemical imbalance' model fails to accommodate any of the facts, beyond the profit requirements of the pharmaceutical companies, but is the unquestioned model accepted by essentially everyone.

A brain with greater density is unnecessary. Human beings are estimated generally to only use 10-15 percent of the capacity of the normal brain. We have no real need of a model predicated on a denser brain. We likewise have no need for a model based on some presumed imbalance of one or two or three chemicals.

The description given above is a Flat Earth version. It is not the actual, final word on the nature of the brain with Turbiasis.

But, just as with the concept of the Earth being flat, it explains some matters, answers some questions and gives us a perspective of such a brain that satisfies us in some of the ways we deal with the questions.

This explanation addresses the differences between chronic depression and situational depression. It covers the frequency of creative thought associated with Turbiasis. It explains why those afflicted may sometimes appear to think more slowly than normal, or more quickly. It can encompass the genetic component that seems so obvious.

It also is an explanation that confers some dignity to Agmina. Seeing oneself as having an evolutionarily more advanced brain, one with greater than normal capacity, might help to shatter the self-image that is inculcated in Agmina when they buy into the stigma. It can, likewise, call into question the slavish acceptance of the stigma by the public at large.

In addition to offering a model that answers some questions and gives some dignity to those sorely in need of it, I have another reason for including a model known to be false. I want to show that it is possible to develop models based on little or no fact and with incorrect analysis that seem reasonable to the lay public and even to most professionals.

Qualified research scientists will see facts and try to formulate a paradigm that incorporates them. But, they then analyze it and test it to see if it stands up. Others will read or hear of the model and accept it, based on the putative authority of the source, or reject it, because it conflicts with their preconceptions. Science demands more than passive acceptance or predisposed conclusions. Having some merit, as this particular model has, is insufficient. It may be used, if there is nothing better, if it has some value but its limitations must be known and acknowledged.

Regardless of that model having several advantages over the 'chemical imbalance' model, we want to understand the problem, as it really is. Given the limitations of our present knowledge and comprehension, we should want to get as close as possible to the truth. We will get there but first I wish to give you some idea of what we are up against.

Chapter 6

Treat or Trick

For a successful technology, reality must take precedence over public relations, for Nature cannot be fooled.
Richard Feynman

The greatest obstacle to discovery is not ignorance - it is the illusion of knowledge.
Daniel J Boorstin

You have heard from the flood of television and print advertisements, the magazine articles and the pronouncements from your physician about the constant flow of progress with reference to the latest and greatest miracle drug.

Ignore all of that. There has been absolutely zero progress in understanding what mental illness is for a considerable number of years. The last increase in understanding it was when it became accepted that it was not caused by demon possession.

It's probably impossible to list the multitude of treatments to which Agmina have been subjected over the years without leaving out something that was, at one time, touted as a miracle.

Water used to be a popular medium. Special dunking chairs were devised. These were used to keep the patient under water until they were on the verge of drowning. They were brought up and revived . . . most of them, anyway.

Wrapping someone as tightly as possible in wet sheets was considered therapeutic. I'm uncertain if it was the water that was supposedly curative or the increased difficulty breathing as the sheets dried that restored one's health. The enthusiasm for treating patients with ice baths of a few hours, or even days, duration finally cooled.

Tables and chairs that violently spun the afflicted were popular for decades. I'm guessing that cleaning up afterward was a drawback.

Beating led the hit parade for generations. Some physicians were more particular than others. Some used only lashes. Others apparently felt that any device was therapeutic, as long as the patient could be rendered senseless.

Lobotomies were all the rage in the 1930s, 40s and 50s. All one needed to do to set things straight in this most complex of organs was to stick a large knitting needle into the patient's brain and wiggle it for a couple of minutes. Check that. It might have been jiggle, instead of wiggle.

Insulin shock treatment had a relatively long day in the sun as the psychiatric flavor of the month. It was quite popular around the time I was born.

Removing teeth was claimed as a cure. The physician who dreamed that up later sought even better results by including several minor organs on the list of unnecessary parts. Each addition naturally was accompanied by the claim of improved outcomes.

When others were unable to duplicate the results of dental therapy, someone figured they might have better luck starting at the other end of the torso. This brilliant physician had a small following dedicated to relief of Turbiasis by relieving patients of their testicles.

But, once again we find a problem: discrimination against women. I assume that they were incapable of being cured.

While I have dealt with it lightly, the reality of how Agmina have been treated in centuries past and, indeed, in the very present times is no joking matter. It is difficult to grasp how not just an errant few but essentially an entire profession could not simply condone and practice such barbarities but congratulate themselves on the humanity and ethics of their calling.

Even those who reluctantly admit to the cruelties of the past, staunchly defend current practices as the latest and greatest in humane, scientific treatments. Some may argue that my flip approach is inappropriate but there is no denying that, from the earliest days to the present, the profession is fully deserving of whatever ridicule and scorn they engender.

Those therapies mentioned above have faded from fashion for the most part but the following are championed as the culmination of enlightenment as practiced by the chosen, the high priests of science and sensibility. But first, permit me to offer my own new therapy.

Another Miracle

It may be an unwritten rule but it appears to be an actual written requirement, fully codified, that every new treatment for Turbiasis must be designated a miracle. I am not disposed to violate such a widely accepted dictum.

Long before I delved into the history of neuroleptics I had gradually come to the conclusion that they were, in my personally favorite terms, 'chemical straitjackets' and 'chemical baby sitters.' I was apparently not the first to describe them so but I learned that many others had used terms no more flattering. Walter Freeman and other researchers and practitioners in the early- and mid-fifties characterized chlorpromazine as a 'chemical lobotomy.' There is a degree of difference between my use and theirs, however. They used such language in a laudatory sense.

Chlorpromazine (Thorazine, *et al.*) belongs to a class of chemicals called phenothiazines. Prior to becoming a miracle this class of compounds was used for more prosaic purposes. Synthetic dyes, antihistamines, anti-emetics and insecticides were based on this group.

As with all miracle treatments, early users and researchers found neuroleptics a valued therapy for a broad range of maladies. The list included schizophrenia, manic states, depression, paranoia, severe anxiety, phobias, Parkinson's (truly ironic), sedation to reduce or eliminate the need for anaesthetics during surgery, obsessions, extreme agitation, senility, epilepsy, and halitosis.

Strangely, other researchers found no efficacy for most of these issues. Perhaps it was just a phase that many miracles must manage to muddle through before the marketing team focuses their resources. Such is the fate of a miracle.

Eventually, it was decided that schizophrenics were the ones most benefitted by this latest miracle. In 1964 a major study sponsored by the National Institute of Mental Health showed 95 percent of those with schizophrenia were improved by neuroleptics and there were no adverse outcomes. This study was a complete farce. It was done on behalf of the drug companies.

There absolutely was no science involved. There could not have been. These were just absurd assertions pulled out of thin air.

The drug companies were not making claims anywhere near 95 percent. No known actual scientific study of neuroleptics has ever shown no adverse outcomes. Among other problems, studies on patients with schizophrenia showed that those treated with neuroleptics had far longer hospital stays and higher rates of relapse.

Companies are prohibited by the FDA from making claims they can't substantiate with studies. They do, of course, make baseless claims but even they would not stretch the percentages that far. Here we see the NIMH doing for the drug companies that which the FDA will not permit them to do for themselves.

It isn't just a bad apple here and another there. It isn't just a rogue company now and then. It isn't corruption in an individual, a company, even an industry. The entire system is corrupt.

Both before and after this NIMH study neuroleptics were found to cause Parkinsonism, tardive dyskinesia, akinesia, akathisia, extrapyramidal disorders, neuroleptic-induced deficit syndrome, neuroleptic malignant syndrome and death among other things. So, according to the NIMH, none of the above maladies are bad for you . . . if you are schizophrenic.

Neuroleptics didn't cure schizophrenia. By dampening the central motor control system it reduced hallucinations but failed to eliminate them. It quieted but did not still the voices. It generally did reduce agitated behavior but patients commonly experienced feelings of intense internal agitation.

Among all of these problems though, I discovered the real benefit of neuroleptics. It was well-hidden but, with tremendous effort and persistence, I was able to ferret out the true nature of this miracle. Neuroleptics quieted the patients. It made them easier for the providers to manage, control and endure. The real role of neuroleptics was as a babysitting aid. It made the life of those who had to be around schizophrenic patients much, much easier. Who could ask for more? It was a true psychiatric miracle.

Once I realized the true value of neuroleptics, I sought to discover if there was a possible alternative, one that might be cheaper, or quicker acting, or more convenient, or more reliable or some combination of these traits. All this putative therapy had to do was calm these patients and offer some advantage over neuroleptics.

Then it hit me, all of a sudden. If I hit someone upside the head with sufficient force, calm would ensue. But what would be the instrument of choice? Many objects came to mind but some might have so little stunning effect that the provider of the therapy is put in jeopardy of retaliation by the patient. The striking area of a ball-peen hammer or a baseball bat would be relatively small or too focused and might too easily cause excessive fracturing of the skull.

After considerable thought and evaluation of a large number of possible instruments, it came to me that, short of designing a tool specifically for the purpose, the ideal would be a skillet. In order to ensure a minimum of confusion, I have foresworn the usual tendency to obfuscate and impress with a strained label. I could have used something on the order of biogenic external assaultive therapy (BEAT) but finally decided to term it simply 'Skillet Therapy.'

The first aspect of researching this was to design the study. I initially had a problem in establishing a control. Other than comparing the treated patients with a group that received a sugar pill and was spared being hit, I could not figure out what to use as a placebo for this purpose.

The answer came hard but I eventually developed an appropriate control. If schizophrenics were seen as abnormal, it made sense to compare the effects of this therapy on them with the effects of this therapy on normal people. But, how to define and find normality?

As the diagnosis of this abnormality of schizophrenia was the purview of physicians, they therefore must be able to recognize normality, as well. That is not to say they themselves are necessarily normal; just that they are able to spot it, if they see it.

Each selected physician would be required to announce their own status — normal or schizophrenic. This would provide the initial study participants. The likelihood is that a majority of the physicians will find themselves to qualify for this control group of normal. The subject group will be formed from their designated patients.

Realizing that there may be other problems which might be alleviated or cured by this therapy, it seemed a good idea to broaden the study. After all, every new product that issues forth from the drug industry is efficacious for at least a dozen or two discrete maladies, whether anyone has heard of them before or not. This would also make the study more cost effective; always a consideration I am told.

In trying to select this third group for the study, I felt the treatment might best work on some specific personality disorders. The study will focus on avarice, prevarication and the absence of empathy. The selection of this particular combination of personality disorders was fortuitous. It has been shown that there is an extremely high incidence of all three of these disorders in an easily identified and homogenous subset of the population. This group is highly concentrated in the executive offices of pharmaceutical companies and health maintenance organizations, particularly so in their marketing departments. Each of these groups will receive identical therapy. Politicians fit the same profile but we could not afford them.

The study must determine and compare the efficacy of several variables. Should the skillets be of cast iron, aluminum or stainless steel? How do copper-bottom skillets compare with those of single materials? Is Teflon coating beneficial? Does striking one on the right side of the head or the left, improve the results? Would it be the same for left-handed people? Does size matter? Should the skillet be heated first?

What should be the number of strikes per session? How frequent should these sessions be? At what point should the frequency be reduced to effect a maintenance level? Must one remain on this regimen on a permanent basis?

I suspect that once word of this promising therapy leaks out, unscrupulous competitors will try to jump in, so a few warnings are necessary. First, don't try this at home. Make certain that the subjects' hair styles do not cushion the blows. Glasses, contacts, hearing aids and false teeth should be removed prior to treatment. Practice makes perfect — door-to-door salesmen are often available.

We have found it preferable to always strike with the bottom of the skillet. The results are too variable otherwise and generally less effective.

The cable television Food Channel is able to provide constant supervision with their experts. Once the testing is complete, the results of the study can then be submitted to the Department of Agriculture for certification A peer-reviewed abstract can be published in *Modern Frying Magazine* and *Reader's Digest*.

Health maintenance organizations will be keeping tabs on the research as skillets are reusable and most physicians will need only one or a small set. We expect this to significantly reduce treatment costs for schizophrenia.

One other discovery I made while doing the preliminary research for this study was stunning. New therapies are a potential source of large amounts of money. This may be part of the motivation for pharmaceutical companies.

In order to generate greater profits, there will be the formation of a cabal, or association, of ethical manufacturers of cooking utensils. Tee-shirts and bobblehead dolls may prove popular. Another possible source of revenue again involves the Food Channel. We are already working to produce a reality show based on schizophrenia. It should be a fun show.

The start of this research unfortunately was delayed for a considerable time. At one point in the grant application there was a reference to this therapy resulting in a Way to Manage the Demented. It was a most unfortunate choice of initials. Our entire staff was quickly escorted by the FBI on a short vacation to Guantanamo Bay.

We are gratified and optimistic, however. From preliminary findings it seems that it will all pan out.

I'm Shocked

Once upon a time there was a medical miracle called Shock Therapy. But, not everyone believes in miracles. These few unbelievers told anyone who would listen that shock therapy was not a miracle. They told others that the Big Bad Wolf was using it to hurt sick people . . . and eating their grandmas.

This caused problems for Mr. Wolf. It cost him money. It inconvenienced him. It made him look like a villain.

Mr. Wolf and his colleagues had to find a way to stop these lies. They huffed and puffed but these unbelievers just wouldn't stop. These unbelievers even made a movie showing the public what shock therapy looked like. The public found it electrifying. Something had to be done.

Once they put their minds to it, Mr. Wolf and his friends found a way to make shock therapy look kinder and gentler. They would give the patients a tranquilizer and a muscle relaxant.

A little toe twitching didn't look all that bad. They even changed the name of the miracle. Now it was electro-convulsive therapy. The acronym, ECT, sounded even more benign. The miracle was refined. And they all lived happily ever after.

Well, not all. The unbelievers still ranted and raved. They claimed that the damage done to the brain wasn't eliminated by preventing the muscles from causing the patient to flop around. Ignore such nonsense. Mr. Wolf and his friends could now show everyone a nice, quiet, well-behaved patient twitching his toes.

ECT induces changes very close to severe concussions. There is hemorrhaging. There is disorientation. There is memory loss. There is incontinence. Autopsies of patients receiving multiple ECT treatments have described areas of devastation. Some had large areas characterized as undifferentiated mush. What's not to like? It is certainly easier on the staff to deal with patients who are either too fearful to act up or unable to do so.

'Oh, but it's not like that anymore,' they say. There have been cosmetic changes since Jack Nickolson got on the wrong side of Louise Fletcher in *One Flew Over the Cuckoo's Nest*. Now they give you muscle relaxants and sedatives. They had to. It was disturbing many of the staff just to watch. The convulsions brought on by ECT were so violent that around 40 percent of the patients in some studies, ended up with broken bones, even a few broken backs.

So, it's much better in these modern, high-tech days with all the compassionate Mildred Ratcheds and HMOs. Now, all the staff sees are a few toes twitching. It's much easier to watch. Just ignore the fact that the muscle relaxants don't ameliorate the mush-making, don't maintain your memories, don't leave you less dependent on Depends. If you would allow me to adjust your delicate, complicated Rolex by using it to replace the key in Benjamin Franklin's kite experiment, then ECT is just your ticket.

If the people who are willing to inflict this on other human beings knew enough about the brain to explain what happens inside the brain when it attempts to absorb such a stunning assault, I would be more than happy to listen. If they could tell me how the brain functions better as mush, I would be interested in learning how that works. If they could tell me why patients receiving ECT experience higher rates of relapse but are better for it, I would put off installing an 8-track tape player in my Yugo and listen.

The sad fact is that they can't answer any of these questions or any of a hundred more I could ask about the brain. They can and will quote studies based on falsified numbers and spurious analysis, however.

After World War II, the International Red Cross judged that prisoners subjected to the "pseudo-medical" abuse of ECT should be compensated. Despite that, a dearth of intellect, imagination and compassion has led to the resurgence of ECT.

If anyone outside the psychiatric profession sent a stunning surge of electricity through the brain of someone strolling through a park, someone not classified as a psychiatric patient, they would open themselves to a criminal charge of aggravated assault or attempted murder. They probably would be committed because a judge or jury would consider it so outlandish an act that the person must be insane. Ironically, they might be sent to a psychiatric hospital. Deciding who is insane and who has diminished capacity becomes more difficult all the time.

Chapter 7

Sweet Little Lies

A lie told often enough becomes truth.
Lenin (Vladimir Ulyanov)

Ye shall know the truth, and the truth shall make you mad.
Aldous Huxley

I don't give them hell. I just tell the truth and they think it is hell.
Harry S. Truman

People who cannot recognize a palpable absurdity are very much in the way of civilization.
Agnes Repplier

Did you notice? I have hinted that the 'chemical imbalance' theory is incorrect. Am I really serious. How could I say such a thing?

Everyone knows it is the cause, or at least the explanation, of Turbiasis. Should I tell you why I make such a rash statement? I should. I will.

We may not know whether the chicken or the egg came first but we do know that the theory, in this case came after the pharmaceutical companies had some results they wanted. They were looking for an explanation that might help them develop more drugs. While they had results they wanted, that in no way means they had results that benefitted the patients.

The 'chemical imbalance' model should really be considered a marketing gimmick. It should also be treated as stumbling block to any understanding of Turbiasis. It is a problem not so much because it is incorrect but because it is believed by so many to be correct.

Who believes it is correct? I am tempted to say everyone. That isn't far from the truth. The general public believes it is correct. Why? That is the only model they have heard about and they heard that it is true from essentially every quarter. The people they trust have told them so.

Essentially all physicians believe it to be true. Whatever their specialty, psychiatry, primary care or podiatry, they have accepted it as fact. Why physicians would trust a pharmaceutical salesman is just one of those imponderables that defies common sense. Almost all Agmina believe it to be true. That is what the high priests of Turbiasis have told them.

Neuroscientists in areas other than those dealing with psychiatric disorders believe it to be true. Since everyone else seems to have faith in that answer and it is not their specialty, they think they are deferring to another specialty and accept what everyone has been told. There is insufficient cross-fertilization between the specialized areas.

That leaves only those neuroscientists working on the problem. Do they believe it to be true? No. They know that it isn't true. They know that it can't be true. I do feel a need to qualify this slightly.

There are researchers working in this field who support the 'chemical imbalance' model. Why? Because they are paid to support it. They are the hacks whose bread is buttered by the pharmaceutical companies. Whether they in fact believe it or not is in doubt. Sinclair Lewis told us, "It is difficult to get a man to understand something when his salary depends upon his not understanding it."

Would these companies really be so craven, so dishonorable, so contemptible? Count out thirteen billion dollars in ones and get back to me. That is a considerable amount of inducement to slant the marketing to their advantage. As impressive an amount as that may be to you and me, that is for only one year in the United States alone. If the rewards for lying are so great, it is understandable that, in certain circles, there is little interest in killing that golden goose.

It is necessary to clarify a certain matter before going further. At times I will say kind things about researchers. At times I will say unkind things about researchers. Actually, it is easy to keep it straight while reading this. There are true researchers. They are trained scientists. Although there are many, they are in the minority in this field. If you see a word of praise for researchers, you may be sure this is the group to which I am referring.

The others are not trained in the art and science of research. They are usually clinical physicians, clinical psychiatrists and too large a percentage of academic psychiatrists. They may be drawn to research as a way to supplement their income. Psychiatry is among the lowest paid specialties. Academia alone seldom provides sufficient income to support a lifestyle that Donald Trump would envy.

They may be drawn into it for the prestige of having a paper published under their name. Whatever the reason, and despite their self-image, they are not qualified scientists.

That is why the pharmaceutical companies pay them so handsomely, because they don't know what they are doing or don't care. The companies can give them the protocols, provide the subjects, do the study and even write the paper. These researchers can become involved at any point after the mold is set, set to provide the desired results.

Some do nothing more than allow the companies to use their names. They have no real involvement in the study.

Selling your soul is a fast track to a pot of gold. If you see words of derision and condescension directed at researchers, you may rest assured it is this type I have in mind.

A recent Harvard study elicited admissions from medical schools across the country that they would allow drug companies to draft articles for medical journals and many would permit them to supply the actual results. Some claim they would not sign a contract to suppress negative results but that is, in reality, a meaningless reservation.

Pharmaceutical companies pay for these studies and therefore own them. They have sued researchers, schools and even government agencies to maintain the secrecy of inconvenient results.

Three-quarters of the medical schools reported clashes over payments after a contract was finalized. Seventeen percent had difficulty in gaining access to the data.

That should not be surprising. The drug industry's trade group clearly claims that the companies own the information and have the exclusive right to determine who may have access to it.

Even though such experiences would make most people wary of dealing with them, the schools' appetites for money exceed whatever qualms they may have. In the medical industry greed triumphs once again. They swallow their pride and ethics, if any, in order to not alienate the golden goose.

A disturbing development began in the 1980s. It was a totally new industry. It runs clinical trials for profit. Any results a pharmaceutical company wants, it can get.

To consider their work scientific is laughable. To consider their output to be honest and factual should be unthinkable. To expect them to have any familiarity with ethics would justify people judging your intelligence quotient to be commensurate with your shoe size. It is unconscionable that the government would allow them to exist, much less that the FDA would accept their trial reports.

The drug industry has taken another tack of late. More and more drug trials are being done overseas, with some companies having passed the fifty percent mark. Perhaps because they deem their profit margins to be inadequate, they claim the reason for this ongoing trend is because these foreign trials can be done more cheaply.

The opportunity to distance themselves from oversight and have a ready excuse for all-expenses paid congressional vacatio . . . er, fact-finding trips could not be considerations to these fine, upstanding exemplars of propriety.

The 'chemical imbalance' model came into being about half of a century ago. It was not well thought out and soon recognized as such. It was really just a wild guess based on an extremely primitive and inaccurate body of knowledge.

They had a drug. They were getting some results that they wanted. They thought that, rather than accidently come upon more and better drugs, as had been the case with this one, it would be nice to know how and why it worked.

It's hard to develop a valid theory of how something works if it doesn't work. But, you say, they were getting results. True, but they would have gotten some kind of results with arsenic, or whiskey, or Ex-lax. Again, they were getting some results they wanted.

So, what was the drug? The drug was chlorpromazine. It was first marketed in the United States as Thorazine. It was developed in France from phenothiazines, a class of chemicals that had been used as anti-emetics, insecticides, synthetic dyes and a few other odds and ends. To this day, half a century later, it has no known effect that cures, alleviates or improves any form of Turbiasis.

So, what were the results? What they wanted was something that would make people with schizophrenia easier to deal with, easier to control. Isn't that a positive outcome? Yes, for those working with these patients.

But, since when has it been considered ethical to medicate or otherwise treat someone else for your benefit? It has been considered ethical ever since the medical community started treating Turbiasis. I have tried but cannot name any other illness where one person takes a medication for another person's problem.

Their problem, the psychiatric hospital physicians and their little helpers, was that it was unpleasant being around schizophrenia. Apparently they never considered how unpleasant is was to have the disease; nor did they consider real people forced to experience the side effects of the drugs. The psychiatrists praised Thorazine as a chemical lobotomy.

They gave a name to the most obvious side effect of the medication. They called it the Thorazine shuffle. It is an artificially induced stupor that reminds one of the behavior of zombies. The image the general public has of schizophrenia is not from seeing the effects of the disease. Their image is actually based on the effects of the medication.

Thorazine and its chemical brethren are classified as neuroleptics.

The priorities demonstrated above are neither new nor rare. They led, and continue to lead, to treatment of schizophrenic patients that is unbelievably inhumane.

I will not dwell here on the disgraceful history of the treatment of people with schizophrenia or Turbiasis in general. I would encourage you to read a very interesting and readable book on the subject by the award-winning journalist Robert Whitaker. The title is, *Mad in America.*

You probably aren't interested in earning a graduate degree in psychopharmacology or neurobiology and I no longer confer such degrees. I think it necessary, however, to provide you with a modicum of scientific understanding of what neuroleptics do.

Neuroleptics shut down or kill dopamine receptors. The effect of shutting these receptors down is to dampen the central motor control system of the brain. The result of this is seen in what is commonly termed the zombie-like state. The observable effects of the dampening of this system are very obvious. There is reduced control of major body movements. That explains the shuffle. There is also drooling. Again, you are seeing the results of reduced motor control. There are other, less noticeable effects but it is hardly an appealing sight or experience.

These are some of the immediate effects. There are longer term effects, some readily observable, some not. These longer term effects are numerous and serious. Some can lead to death. The best known of these effects is tardive dyskinesia. Just a few months on a neuroleptic, or sometimes less, can bring on this problem.

It seems that the most common symptom of tardive dyskinesia is a pronounced tic, usually a facial tic but it could be a contortion of the face. Others may develop uncontrollable movements of the limbs. Still others may involuntarily stick out their tongues, frequently and for extended periods of time. Tardive dyskinesia can cause problems with standing and walking, eating and swallowing. Intelligible speech can become impossible.

Associated with tardive dyskinesia is a diminished intellectual functioning. As if that were not sufficient, it is also associated with behavioral problems.

About half of those with tardive dyskinesia are unaware they have it. It causes one to lose the ability to know their own condition.

Autopsies reveal damage caused by neuroleptics. The problem is that no one particular type of damage is found to be universal. The type of damage varies from individual to individual. It seems obvious that people with schizophrenia have been subjected to powerful drugs that are toxic in numerous, unpredictable ways.

It is unconscionable that physicians prescribe these potent toxins with no understanding of what they do or how they do it and no regard for their patients. They are fond of seeing themselves as scientists, as healers, as ethical, as caring. The only honest response that seems appropriate is: *bullshit!*

There may be cases of people who develop tardive dyskinesia and recover from it. I have heard the claim in informal discussions that remission has happened but I am personally unaware of any cases and find nothing credible in the literature that characterizes it as temporary or reversible. Basically, if you get it, you got it. It is a permanent condition.

In dosage levels that are common in the United States, seventy to ninety percent of the dopamine receptors become incapacitated or killed. This just happens to be in the same range as what happens naturally in some people. The people to whom this happens naturally are diagnosed as having Parkinson's Disease. One of the outcomes of using neuroleptics is an artificially induced Parkinson's Disease. It even has its own term: Parkinsonism.

If you get the chance, ask someone with Parkinson's if they think what they have should be considered an acceptable side effect for someone with another serious disease. Ask them if they think that it is ethical and justifiable to induce it into someone just so the physician's, nurse's, social worker's and family member's time spent around a person with schizophrenia will be less bothersome.

If you don't know anyone with Parkinson's Disease, write to Michael J. Fox or Muhammad Ali. By the way, there were studies that claimed neuroleptics to be efficacious for the treatment of Parkinson's.

All of the side effects are worthy of explication but there are two that beg for mention: akathisia and akinesia. The first is the one you should worry about most. Akathisia causes extreme inner anxiety. You may ask why that should be of any concern to one not taking a neuroleptic. Should you be worried about a patient who is very fidgety, constantly pacing or showing other such behaviors? The simple answer is yes. This is merely the visible expression of the agony, pain, anguish and torment that you can not see.

Your problem is that, in a very significant percentage of the people trying to deal with akathisia, a couple of other expressions of this are aggression and violence. It appears that not only is akathisia a side effect of neuroleptics but abrupt withdrawal of the drugs can also trigger it. When the media plays up a story of murder or other serious violent acts by one with schizophrenia, the odds are heavy that akathisia is involved. Again, we are not seeing schizophrenic behavior. We are seeing drug-induced behavior.

Akinesia may be less of a danger to those not taking neuroleptics than akathisia but it represents a desperate situation for those who are. It may express itself in temporary paralysis and/or in extremely deadened emotions. The former may be easier for an unaffected person to grasp, if not fully appreciate. The latter may not seem even to be a problem to the patient in a given situation simply because of the deadening of the emotions. One's reaction to a tragedy, personal or other, will be inappropriate. One experiences no pleasure. As with other aspects of Turbiasis, it is easy to write a simple description but impossible to convey the reality.

Throughout my research I found a far too common, constant and consistent response to these side effects. When faced with various side effects caused by these medications, physicians overwhelmingly react with the same tendency. More. Their answer to every problem is to increase the dosage.

They know the drugs are powerful. They know what the side effects are. By definition the drugs cause the side effects and yet, even when the side effects are potentially life threatening, their solution is all too commonly: more. Perhaps it is simply a reflection of the seemingly innate American credo: more is better.

Perhaps you disagree with my characterization that neuroleptics are used to make patients more bearable to be around. Then you would be well-advised to read some of the medical papers from the 1950s when it was introduced. You might even want to read the advertising and the marketing materials sent to psychiatric hospitals. The emphasis was heavily slanted to how the drugs made the patients easier to handle and control. Nothing has changed. That is still the emphasis. The materials are merely somewhat more discreet now but the message is the same.

I would be remiss if I failed to mention the only other marketing point. We have covered the fact that those with schizophrenia are often unpleasant to be around. By putting patients in a semi-comatose state, it was not only easier for the professionals to deal with, it was easier also for the families. This coincided nicely with the beginning of the efforts in the mid-1960s to save money by reducing the populations of patients in psychiatric hospitals.

To some extent the 'calming' effects of these drugs made people think deinstitutionalization was feasible. Just send the zombies home or to the community. The fact that they were able to release so many patients was touted as proof of the efficacy of these miracle drugs. You may see the results of emptying the psychiatric hospitals in the jails and prisons and sleeping on the streets in your local downtown.

Missing were any stories of people being cured, going back to the life that had been interrupted. Missing were testimonials from patients of how much better they felt. There were claims of patients making miraculous recoveries. There were claims. There just were not any verified stories of real individuals.

You may be thinking that I am telling only part of the story. I am. You may be thinking that I am omitting the positive aspects of neuroleptics. I will now provide you with what are boasted to be the positives, aside from those benefits for the staff and drug companies.

Hallucinations are sometimes less vivid. Voices are sometimes less intrusive. That's it. That's all the additional benefits they can claim. The hallucinations don't go away, neither do the voices. They sometimes lose some intensity. "Isn't that good or at least sufficient?" you ask. I'm not going to make that decision for someone else. I'm certainly not inclined to force such dangerous and damaging drugs on anyone or lie to anyone in an effort to cajole anyone into taking them 'voluntarily.' Those are the ways most people start taking neuroleptics.

Studies have shown well over eighty percent of people taking neuroleptics for a long term (six months to a year or longer) being beset with one or more of the serious side effects. Estimates range from thirty percent to two-thirds of those taking the drugs as not responding. Not responding means to them that the physicians, nurses, *et al.* don't get their benefits.

A side note is also interesting. One of the two French physicians who developed and promoted neuroleptics made a visit to North America for a lecture engagement. He was surprised at the way it was being used here. The common dosages here were up to fifty times that used in Europe. Over there a study using levels reduced from those lower levels already common in Europe showed better results. If using less improves the results, it is not too farfetched to think that their elimination might also show some benefits. *C'est la mort.*

While there is a dampening of the visible, physical restlessness and agitation with the administration of neuroleptics, patients describe an inner, emotional agitation. Most, in my experience, will aver that the inner agitation is far, far more troubling and disconcerting than the physical agitation. There is also a feeling of separation from oneself. That last sentence is very simple and straightforward but it doesn't convey the emotional impact, the horror of losing touch with your own self.

Taking neuroleptics has at least one other major consequence. Studies, both here and abroad, have shown that taking this family of medications for even a short period increases the likelihood of relapse by a factor of three to ten times. What is a short period? Different studies used differing definitions but, generally, one could use a period of from a couple of weeks to six months.

I may repeat it elsewhere in speaking of drugs used to treat other forms of Turbiasis but this significant increase in relapse is not restricted to neuroleptics. Studies have shown this effect with such a number of brands of antidepressants and other psychopharmaceuticals that it is probably true of all. I have found no study of any of them that demonstrates otherwise concerning this disturbing problem.

Two countries had the distinction of being, far and away, the leading users of neuroleptics: the United States and the former Soviet Union. This caused a problem for the Congress. Dissidents from the Soviet Union began getting out horror stories of torture to the outside world. Congress was waiting with baited breath to find another stick with which to beat those terrible communists (such was always good for a few more votes with no downside and minimal costs).

The stories were gruesome. They detailed some of the methods of torture. It appears that one of the favorites (of the guards, not the prisoners) was the administration of neuroleptics. This was also one of the most feared (by the prisoners, not the guards).

How could these masters of evil be so heartless as to employ such depraved methods on helpless human beings? Whoops! Weren't we using the very same drugs on ill, helpless people here in the good ole U.S. of A.? Weren't congressmen taking sizeable sums of money from pharmaceutical makers to push this on their constituents?

The World Health Organization, researchers in Finland and several others, here in the United States and elsewhere, have found other therapies far superior to anti-psychotics. But, American medicine insists on using treatments that demonstrably harm the patients and don't improve their lives or cure them. Why?

Before leaving neuroleptics to look at other classes of drugs used on Agmina, let me list some, not all, of the problems they cause: akathisia, akinesia, blunted emotions, neuroleptic malignant syndrome, neuroleptic-induced deficit syndrome, extrapyramidal symptoms, blindness, fatal blood clots, arrhythmia, heat stroke, swollen breasts, impotence, obesity, sexual dysfunction, blood disorders, painful skin rashes, seizures, having children with birth defects, reduced learning ability, reduced motor skills and reduced problem solving ability. Being generic, it's very inexpensive now. Could I interest you in trying it?

Neuroleptics, under that name, have been used somewhat less in the past decade plus. The reason is the introduction of a new medication for schizophrenia. I use the word new with considerable reservations. The pharmaceutical treatment of all forms of Turbiasis has depended on four groups of medications. All four came to us around the middle of the last century. They have tinkered with these basic groups and played games in the marketing of them but there remain only four.

Neuroleptics were first claimed to treat everything, save the mange, but they finally settled on schizophrenia. That enlightened decade also gave us tricyclics, monoamine oxidase inhibitors and lithium. There may be some who object that my claim is dated. What about selective serotonin reuptake inhibitors (SSRIs) and atypicals?

The former do the same thing as tricyclics. There may be some minor chemical manipulations and a new name and marketing campaign but they accomplish the same thing. They block the neurotransmitters from being absorbed back into the neuron (reuptake). In fact, SSRIs are a subclass of tricyclics. They are tricyclics.

The use of the term selective is very misleading. They affect other neurotransmitters as well as serotonin. They are named as though different chemical classes but that is a distinction without difference. Some physicians may object but to me it's the difference between a car wreck and a train wreck. You don't want to be involved with either.

Next we come to atypicals. These really just combine dampening down the dopamine receptors using neuroleptics conflated with an antidepressant. Clozapine led the way. When it was first available, it was widely known to have a considerable potential for killing you.

The FDA required everyone taking it to have periodic blood tests. The manufacturer imposed the restriction that only a certain chain of labs be used for these tests. It should surprise no one that this particular manufacturer had a very healthy financial stake in that particular chain. The cost of the combination of drug and tests brought the annual bill to the neighborhood of $9,000 per patient.

Sufficient outrage was expressed when the financial link became known that the company had to spread some of the laboratory work around to others. It wasn't as though this test was rare or that it required esoteric technology or special equipment.

It was a routine test. They just wanted more money from those suffering from schizophrenia or from you, in insurance premiums or taxes. They weren't particular where they got it from.

Competition in the testing brought the cost down below $4,000 *per annum*. This reduction in costs needs to be compared with the costs of neuroleptics and tricyclics, which have been generic for a very long time. That was the impetus for developing atypicals. There was insufficient profit in a product that was at that time approaching four decades on the shelves and costing less than ten dollars a month.

And you probably thought their interest was in finding a better treatment for Agmina. Wasn't an atypical better than a neuroleptic? Wasn't a thirty-fold increase in costs justified by the improvement?

Despite all of the marketing campaigns, an atypical was, according to all of the studies independent of the drug manufacturers and the FDA, no more effective than those old neuroleptics. Competing products came out and reduced, not eliminated, the danger of the pioneer atypical but still have failed to prove any more effective.

The claim of reducing certain side effects of neuroleptics is problematical. There may be some reduction of tardive dyskinesia but not provably, consistently and significantly. Others claimed the reduction was to extrapyramidal symptoms. I think you are allowed to take your pick. Whether there is any reduction of a couple of side effects, by using a combination of two types of drugs with differing known side effects, you shouldn't be surprised if you get a greater number of side effects than from either one alone.

Atypicals were studied but dropped fifteen years earlier. The reason? They were considered too dangerous. Given the dangers of the basic neuroleptics, one wonders how dangerous atypicals are to be considered too dangerous.

I gave more time than intended to neuroleptics but it does show how this concentration on drugging people got started. Anyway, the starting point for the 'chemical imbalance' model was based on having produced results that were seen as desirable. Despite claims made to the patients and public, there was never any consideration of the patients' cure, improvement or well-being. It is not possible to start from the point of how to successfully dampen one's central motor system, completely disregard the patients' problems and arrive at an understanding of what Turbiasis is, what causes it or how to treat it.

When looking for a theory, what they found was mentioned above. Dopamine receptors were shut down. Since this gave them the results they wanted, it was easy to postulate that the problem was caused by too much dopamine. *Voila,* too much of a chemical meant there was an imbalance. This theory ignores a few minor points. In about the same time frame (three to six weeks) as it takes to have an effect, the brain has deployed its defenses, in one way by growing new receptors. Also, the neurons have increased their firing rates.

The original claims were that the neuroleptics worked by shutting down the D2 and D3 receptors. But others had the results they wanted that had only a negligible effect on those two receptor types. Some people with schizophrenia had higher levels of dopamine than normal; some had lower. Some had normal levels. Whoops. So did people without schizophrenia.

There was the rare voice crying out in the wilderness, objecting to this nonsense, but science has proven that dollar signs are one of the most effective noise suppressing agents in the universe. The drug lords have sufficient dollar signs to muffle the Big Bang.

This new theory of how neuroleptics worked proved so attractive (read profitable) that the other accidental drug classes used it too. All they had to do was determine what chemical was affected by the drug they had and claim that an imbalance of that chemical was the problem.

The tricyclic and monoamine oxidase inhibitors worked on the monoamines, primarily dopamine, serotonin and norepinephrine. They increased the availability of the monoamines, so that meant that without these miracle drugs there was a deficit. Just as with an excess, a deficit qualifies as an imbalance. See how well it all worked out?

Okay, so we already know that neuroleptics don't address the problem of schizophrenia, only the problem of being around someone with it. They do harm. They take people who are desperately ill and make them feel worse and make them worse. They can permanently disable or kill. Although they temporarily change the level of activity of dopamine, there was not necessarily any imbalance to correct. How do we know? Autopsies.

Those who had taken these drugs actually had grown new dopamine receptors, as the body and brain tried to adapt to the damage. Of those who had not been medicated, some had above average levels of dopamine, some had average levels and some had lower than average levels. The same was found in people without schizophrenia. The significance of a dopamine imbalance was first primarily as a guess based on ignorance and then as the foundation for a conscious hoax.

There are two points to make at this juncture. The first is that there are no tests to determine levels of monoamine neurotransmitters, except by autopsy. If anyone tells you that you have a 'chemical imbalance,' they are merely spitting out the party line based on a theory that has been known for at least forty years to be total rubbish, scientific garbage. The best advice available is to absolutely avoid anyone who spouts such nonsense.

The second point is more involved. Reading about the full range of pharmaceuticals, one gets the impression, as is certainly intended, that this industry, as it continues on its inevitable march of scientific progress, is headed towards drugs that are ever more specific; the long-dreamed of Silver Bullets. They don't say so but lack of specificity is what causes side effects.

Whether they are successful in producing more specific products in areas other than those aimed at the psychiatric market, I don't know but that is the direction they tell us they are headed. With that as the established direction for everyone else, they take off in the opposite direction when it comes to those for dealing with Turbiasis.

While on this subject of specificity and Silver Bullets, I should note some reservations on my part. There was a great deal of use of the term 'Silver Bullet' in the 1950s and 1960s. I heard of it frequently and, as everyone else, automatically accepted it as a desirable goal. Now I wonder. Specificity is just a different word for the same concept.

If all, or most all, diseases are complex, involving several elements of the brain and/or body, why should we expect a medication that very selectively effects one chemical compound or one part to address the entire complexity?

I understand that only three or four diseases appear to be caused by a single gene. Turbiasis is not one of them. If we knew enough about the exact and total biological basis for one particular form of one disease, we likely then would need a number of absolutely specific drugs, each aimed at one unique target. So, that would require a clip of several Silver Bullets selected for just one variation of one disease. A different assortment would seem to be needed for other varieties of that disease. Daddy, are we there yet?

I mentioned the combining of two classes of drugs for atypicals. If each class has its own complement of side effects (neither is a Silver Bullet) and you compound them, you are liable to a larger number of side effects. In this particular combination you actually get at least one additional serious side effect that you don't get from either class alone.

The industry is certainly aware of the marketing value of greater specificity. It makes them appear capable of greater precision; therefore, they appear to be more scientifically advanced. Not only do they promote it as the goal but even in psychopharmaceuticals they play the game. The term atypical was carefully chosen. Typical is similar to common. Atypical connotes the uncommon. It conveys an impression of limited, special, rare. They want you to believe that it is more specific while actually being less so. That isn't where they stop. Have you heard of SSRIs (Prozac *et al.*)? The first letter of that acronym stands for selective.

We know that the atypicals are the antithesis of specific. What about the SSRIs? The second letter stands for serotonin. Just what is serotonin? It's a neurotransmitter, you say. Yes, but! Serotonin, as many, perhaps most of the chemicals in the body, is and does several things.

Serotonin initially was used to induce labor. It didn't do that as a neurotransmitter. Serotonin is a primary agent in the clotting of blood. It doesn't do that as a neurotransmitter. Serotonin tightens blood vessels. It doesn't do that as a neurotransmitter. It also increases blood pressure and heart rate. I could list all of the roles that we know serotonin plays but I want to stop and elaborate on these last two.

The reason for focusing on these is because they directly affect me. As for the first one, there's reason for serious doubts that induction of labor would be successful in my case.

I recently had a stent placed in one of my coronary arteries. The reason is because of heart disease. I'm not the only person with a clogged artery. Someone who has heart disease does not need to increase the agent that tightens the blood vessels and clots the blood while raising blood pressure and pulse.

When I mentioned this to a physician, he claimed that Prozac only affected serotonin levels in the brain. Were that true, you would have a degree of specificity. It wouldn't be absolute specificity but it would be well on the way. Was he right? I could not find a single neuroscientist that agreed with his assertion. They were, in fact, adamant that Prozac traveled throughout the body and acted throughout the body.

I also have glaucoma. There are drainage ducts in the eye that are supposed to relieve any buildup of pressure. Pressure damages and eventually will destroy the optic nerve. Any agent that tightens the blood vessels also tightens those ducts. Even antihistamines are off the list of allowed medications for people with glaucoma. They restrict your sinus drainage and as a side effect tighten up the eyes' drainage ducts.

I have never found a psychiatrist or other physician who asks a patient with depression whether they have either glaucoma or heart disease. I have never found a patient who was asked these questions. Why? Either the pharmaceutical salesman didn't mention it to the physician in their 'educational' sessions or he told his student that it has no effect or the physician made it up on the spur of the moment as the only excuse he could muster. Making up facts as needed is a time-honored tradition for defenders of 'chemical imbalance.'

Remember above here where I related a physician saying that Prozac only affected serotonin levels in the brain? You very well may have heard or read something about the serotonin receptor, obviously the counterpart to the serotonin neurotransmitter. I want you to replace the image that conjures with another one. Neurobiologists have identified at least fifteen different types of serotonin receptors, so far. What do they do? We have fairly good guesses about the functions of one, perhaps two.

Just to complicate matters a bit, some of these types of receptors have as many as four subtypes that have been found, to this point. Do you really want to go down to the next level? There is at least one more level.

To get to the bottom of this, we have next to no knowledge of all the possible functions of just this one chemical compound. We absolutely know one specific power it doesn't possess. We know that increasing or decreasing it doesn't improve or degrade depression despite the money and effort spent to convince you so.

For someone lacking any knowledge of how little we know to blithely tell you, based on his/her claimed expertise, that you have an imbalance of a neurotransmitter is to commit a fraud. For someone to tell you that serotonin is the agent that controls your depression is to exhibit their ignorance or commit a fraud.

If you run across someone spouting this nonsense, ask him or her to provide you the results of the tests that show the imbalance. Just be careful if he or she responds by ordering those (postmortem) tests. A safer alternative might be to ask him or her to list all of the serotonin receptor types and subtypes involved, the function of each and on which specific one the drug selectively acts.

Now that we have addressed just how non-selective these selective drugs are with the different functions of serotonin, let's take the next step. Do these selective serotonin drugs limit themselves to serotonin. Don't bet the farm. Every one of these drugs plays upon other compounds. I am not now referring to the fact that there are cascading effects from the initial effect on the serotonin receptors.

These selective medications have direct effects on norepinephrine, dopamine and other compounds. There is no point in elaborating on these but it is important to know that the naming of this subclass of drugs is misleading. This deception was intentional.

I have a problem reconciling the claims of selectivity for these medicines with the claims for their usefulness. SSRIs are widely advertised and prescribed for a host of maladies. Among the problems that we are told they are appropriate for are depression, attention-deficit hyperactivity disorder, obsessive-compulsive disorder, migraine headaches, arthritis, anxiety, social anxiety, losing weight, anorexia, bulimia, stopping smoking, alcoholism, substance abuse, premenstrual syndrome, claustrophobia, fear of flying, hangnail, *etc*. The list seems to get longer every day.

Now, if this drug is so specific, what does it act upon that is not only common to all of these complaints but significant enough a factor to provide relief for all of them? If what it does to these various conditions differs, it is not specific. We know that physicians change medications for patients with depression, for example, because they don't get any results or there are side effects. Often a patient gets a cocktail of drugs prescribed. They are known as human toxic waste dumps.

If a drug does not work on some varieties of depression, are we then to expect this same selective drug (selective for serotonin, the supposed problem causing depression) to work on one or more or all of the other maladies listed above? If we accept them as selective, there is a logical problem. Since they are not selective, as claimed and named, thankfully we have no need to deal with a problem in logic. The fact that they don't help with any of these conditions also helps us avoid having to impose any further logic.

Another little problem is that all of the antidepressants interfere with the neuronal processes which must clear excess neurotransmitters away so that the space is available for the next messenger, one that might be a different chemical, a different message to a different receptor or receptor subtype. Our body or brain may want us to respond differently to a different situation. By interfering with that need, the artificial introduction of chemicals that prevent a necessary response could put the subject in jeopardy.

Not long ago I was taken to the hospital for a suspected heart attack. The reason for such suspicion was that, as mentioned earlier, I had a stent implanted in a coronary artery about six months previously. I was still a smoker at that time. A physician's assistant came by. She asked how I was doing. I replied that I desperately wanted a cigarette. She offered to get me an anti-depressant, not Zyban for some reason, to help me . My response was an emphatic no. She was upset that I was, to her way of thinking, so ignorant of the value of the drug. Let's discuss ignorance of the drug.

The information that accompanies these drugs state that they take three or more weeks to have an affect. I wanted immediate relief from my craving for nicotine. I would be able to smoke upon leaving the hospital. I was there slightly less than forty-eight hours.

My medical history, which she had, mentioned my manic-depression. It didn't indicate that I was taking any medication for the problem but she was a physician's assistant to a cardiology group and the records she had were from the cardiologists. She never asked if I was already taking anti-depressants and, in fact, was unaware of my having this particular malady.

Being a physician's assistant in cardiology, one would hope that she was familiar with the effects of serotonin as it directly related to heart disease: tightening of the arteries, increasing the clotting of the blood. Serotonin and norepinephrine cause changes in blood pressure and heart rate. Significant increases in serotonin can result in tremors and organ failures. Those effects don't take three or more weeks.

I wish that all cardiologists were aware of the attributes of serotonin and their own limitations as regards the subject of Turbiasis and the treatment of it. Also, I would like to think that physicians' assistants didn't feel that their limited training, experience and scope of competence included a far more complex realm of knowledge. This presumption of competence in another field is even more distressing in light of such an amazing deficiency in one's own field. I also wonder why patients must spend all that time filling out questionnaires detailing their entire medical history if the physicians and their assistants ignore them.

Physicians and their assistants get almost all of their pharmaceutical education from detail men, drug salesmen. Is a Prozac salesman going to tell them not to give any of their patients Prozac? How many prescriptions for Prozac would they write? How long would that salesman continue to hold that job? Do cardiologists write prescriptions for anti-depressants? Yes. Why? Because these salesmen lie to them. Should they depend on liars for their education?

I was too angry at the physician's assistant at the time to consider a salient point. A counselor to whom I later related this incident reminded me how fortunate I was. Being upset at the idea of taking an antidepressant is frequently considered sufficient grounds for psychiatric commitment. The power and universality of the acceptance of this hoax is difficult to believe and impossible to exaggerate. Inadvertently, I had put myself in jeopardy for expressing my refusal to be grateful for her ignorance.

It isn't just cardiologists and their assistants. Primary care physicians and a host of other specialties routinely prescribe these medications. Why? First, they really have not the foggiest idea of what they are messing around with; either the brain or the drugs. This makes them easy prey for the drug salesmen. Next, they have an opportunity to make more money.

Giving a pill to someone with Turbiasis makes it easier for the psychiatrist, the social worker, the mental health clinic, the psychiatric hospital, the pharmacological companies — anyone providing treatment to that person. A pill makes the patient easier to be around. A pill helps speed up the process. It requires less time be spent with the patient. That reduced requirement of time gives the provider the opportunity to see a greater number of patients. That then translates into more income. Specialties other than psychiatry are encouraged by the salesmen to jump into this area as a quick and easy way to increase income. We shouldn't be surprised when they do.

I am not concerned with the convenience or bank balances of providers. I could not care less whether they had a good day at the office. To be as honest, direct and nice about it as possible, I don't give a shit. My primary concern is for the person suffering from Turbiasis. That should be true of all providers, also. If it isn't, they should find another line of work, immediately. They should not pass Go. They should not collect $200.

Chapter 8

More Little Lies

One of the most striking differences between a cat and a lie is that a cat has only nine lives.

Mark Twain

Please don't lie to me, unless you're absolutely sure I'll never find out the truth.

Ashleigh Brilliant

That's not a lie, it's a terminological inexactitude.
Also, a tactical misrepresentation.

Alexander Haig

Well, we know that neuroleptics don't even address the problem of schizophrenia, do serious, permanent damage to the body and brain and can kill.

So, do antidepressants work? You saw just above that we haven't the foggiest idea of what these drugs do or what to use them for, beyond generating income for the pharmaceutical companies and physicians.

We have no idea how they function. Perhaps I'm just an old stick-in-the-mud for thinking those are awfully flimsy excuses for spending over $27 billion each and every year and messing around in an organ with which they are unfamiliar. Any congressman worth his purchase price can come up with more creative excuses than that for spending several billion dollars.

Those of you familiar with these medications know that they don't work immediately. You are told that it will be three to four weeks before they begin to have an effect. If you ask why, you will most likely be told that there has to be a sufficient build up of the drug in your system.

What are considered therapeutic dosages are, to the brain, floods of chemicals overwhelming it. Remember, there are many hundreds of millions of active parts and thousands of compounds in that little three-pound organ all carrying out their important work at the cellular level and below. To operations on that scale, milligrams are the equivalent of gallon upon gallon. We rarely see the need to fill up thimbles by flooding them with bathtubs of water daily for weeks. Ignore such nonsense.

Actually, the effects of Prozac, for instance, have begun within a couple of hours. If the theory was correct, that you have a deficiency of serotonin, you should begin feeling better within that same time frame.

The brain has a multitude of feedback systems, for both positive feedback and negative feedback. It, as does the body, tries to maintain a balance. Sometimes these systems work correctly, sometimes not.

Most people are familiar with the interaction of sugar and insulin. You eat a cinnamon roll. Your blood sugar level goes up. You feel energized.

But, your body doesn't want that much sugar. So, insulin kicks in and drives down the blood sugar level. When it drives it down below normal, you have a lack of energy. You are hungry. You may even get the shakes. Your body wants to bring the level up because insulin overcompensated. That is only one of several such mechanisms.

Shortly after Prozac sends your levels up, not making you feel good, a reaction reverses the situation, putting the levels below normal. If the imbalance theory worked, you are now feeling worse than before you took the pill. Thankfully, the theory is wrong.

Placebos

Speaking of sugar, before the FDA will approve a drug, the manufacturer has to show that it works and that it is safe. No, *Cinderella* is another fairy tale. A new drug should be at least as effective as those already on the market and should also be at least as effective as a placebo. Placebos are commonly referred to as sugar pills. Unlike these medications, sugar at these levels has negligible harmful side effects.

The FDA says give us two studies that show the new drug as effective as a placebo. Eli Lilly had to do five studies to get two showing Prozac performed as well as a sugar pill. Their competitors had a more difficult time. They couldn't get two out of five. It took them a few more tries.

Interestingly, the FDA told Eli Lilly that their protocols for the successful tests were biased in favor of the drug. Did the FDA make them do it over again? No. The FDA accepted the results of the studies that they cited as biased and invalid. Were Lilly's offers to FDA staff more attractive than those of their competitors?

With a biased study, Prozac must have really outshone the placebo. Oops! It only showed equivalent results. Unbiased tests have shown the placebo winning by a statistically significant margin.

Do you want more than my word and that of the FDA that the drug companies use biased studies? Okay. How about the word of the drug companies themselves?

Janssen charged Eli Lilly with setting up biased studies. Then, Lilly found Janssen's studies biased. It turns out that both were right. They agreed to refrain from making accurate charges against each other.

While on the subject of placebos, you might find it interesting that they have become significantly more effective over the years. How's that? Sugar is still sugar, isn't it? It sounds odd until you think about it.

A recent study of the effectiveness of placebos was compared to some results in 1980. They indeed have improved. The explanation is simple.

Placebos work for some people when they think they will work. They think they are taking the medication. The brain causes an improvement on its own, without benefit of a drug.

Back in 1980, fewer people had been sold on the idea that drugs were effective. Since that time, the situation has changed. All of the marketing has had its effect. Far more people now believe that these drugs work. As the efficacy of the placebo depends on the subject's belief that it will work, when more believe more experience relief. The placebos, therefore, show an increase in their effectiveness.

What I haven't been able to find is a study that concludes that any presumed benefits from the drugs are really due to the placebo effect.

If you form two groups of a hundred subjects each and give one group the placebo while the other gets a drug and each group has twenty-five subjects reporting positive results, what does that tell you? Researchers assume that the twenty-five in the first group benefitted from the placebo effect. That seems a reasonable inference, as there was no drug involved to credit with the improvement. The other twenty-five are deemed to have benefitted from the drug. Why?

Neither group knew if they were getting the placebo or the drug. Would not the second group have some subjects who experienced the placebo effect? If there were those who experienced it and you added them to the number who actually benefitted from the drug, would you not expect that group to show much higher numbers than the group with only the placebo?

If we assume that the second group had a like number as the first who would benefit from the placebo effect and find that the two groups had equal numbers reporting benefits, we would have to admit that the drug benefitted no one in the study group. We would have to admit that the drug was useless.

Could it be that the drugs only help people who are helped by the placebo effect? Maybe we could save some money by prescribing only sugar pills.

When those taking the placebo are told, their improvement immediately disappears. So far, I have not found a study that reported the results of telling those taking the drug that they were taking a placebo. Some may object that lying to them would be unethical. Many of these same ethical people in other circumstances demonstrate serious ethical lapses.

If temporarily permitting people to think they are taking a drug when taking a placebo is acceptable, why is the reverse unacceptable? Aside from the supposed ethical question, it would help establish whether and to what extent the results ascribed to the drug were, in reality, more properly attributable to the placebo effect. I could be easily convinced that consideration plays a larger role in why it is not done than any ethical considerations. They really do not want to know.

Taking several studies that the FDA did not characterize as biased and subtracting the percentages of people improved through the placebo effect from the percentages imputed to the drug, I ended up with negative numbers. I'm inclined to think that the damage done by the drugs reduces the number that would be helped by the placebo effect.

I understand that at least one reader is still wondering about the FDA's concern for studies comparing a drug with a placebo and how the studies could be biased. For someone who has been on any of these drugs for as long as the manufacturer says is needed to begin feeling the effect, there is a warning. One is admonished not to stop taking the drug abruptly. Stopping abruptly is called a washout and leads to what is known as a rebound.

When your systems have made adjustments in an attempt to accommodate the drug, quick withdrawal creates problems. This is a well-known aspect of street drugs. Going cold turkey with a street drug can be a dreadful experience. Going cold turkey on psychopharmaceuticals also can bring on a great deal of unpleasantness.

Groups picked to be given a placebo in these studies are filled with people who have been taken off a drug abruptly. Is this just a coincidence? I'll let you make up your own mind.

When the drug companies design the studies, they require the placebo subjects to be actively psychotic. They specify that patients dependent on neuroleptics, anti-depressants or whatever, be taken off abruptly.

The problem is that, though they may experience a psychotic episode as a result, they are experiencing drug withdrawal. They may experience both the withdrawal and the psychosis. Though those conducting the study probably will not be able to differentiate between the two, they are not the same. The study design also ignores the differences.

I am again brought back to the question of ethics. Can these people really see themselves as ethical when requiring people with schizophrenia or depression to regress, imposing upon them the pain and trauma of drug withdrawal and putting them into a psychotic state unnecessarily, just to make their dangerous, toxic, destructive products look as good as a sugar pill? Placebos must truly be miracle drugs in order to outperform the wonderful spawn of the drug makers while at such a disadvantage.

Although placebos are colloquially referred to as sugar pills. That is not always accurate. Curiously, many of these studies use very low dosages of the drug being tested as the placebo. I say curiously because it would seem an embarrassment if people knew that a dose of their drug intended to be so small as to be ineffective actually did as well or better than the 'therapeutic' dosage.

Do you really want people that brilliant playing with the innards of your brain? If you have a lot of confidence in the ethical standards of these people, you would have loved the Inquisition and Enron.

The Standard of Ethics

It's really unnecessary for these pretend researchers to play such games. It's far easier to lie about the results. These are honorable people engaged in a humanitarian cause.

Surely they wouldn't invent results just because a wealthy company paid them a considerable sum of money. How could I dare to accuse them of being so vile? Perhaps because it's true and the documentation is both voluminous and undeniable.

Once upon a time, a fairly recent time, an honorable, respected healer became the president of his state's psychiatric association. He also once chaired the committee on ethics. He became involved in a research study. Involved might be too strong a word. He lent his name and credibility to the study and promoted the results. The study was for one of the atypicals.

About half the people in the study did not complete it. That is pretty much the norm. Some studies have rates of sixty percent or greater not finishing. Why? Some cannot tolerate the new drug. Some cannot tolerate the old drug. Some cannot tolerate the withdrawal.

Some commit suicide. In this short study several did so, some while still participating.

What about those that don't complete the trial? Unless the reason is that they committed suicide while active in the trial, we don't know. They just get lost. Suicides, even for those active in a trial, as in this one, commonly go unreported in the study, as it is available to the FDA, medical community and the public.

For those dropping out, the adverse effects they may experience are not reported. Did they commit suicide? It's known that at least one did. None of this will reflect badly on the drug though, so praise the Lord and pass the medication.

Was the drug approved? Yes. How? Well, you see, while the nurses' reports did mention severe problems and suicidal ideation in patients, this paragon of the profession reported absolutely no adverse side effects. In this business lying is no impediment to a reputation as the quintessence of ethical standards.

The pharmaceutical salesmen hand out copies of the glowing report to psychiatrists, general practitioners, anyone with a prescription pad. These physicians may recognize the author's name. They are impressed with his credentials. They are impressed with his credibility. The pharmaceutical company got their money's worth out of him.

The study noted above was carried out among patients in a hospital. Hospitals are supposed to be places where physicians help you. That is the belief of all patients but is commonly inapplicable to those with Turbiasis.

Tilt

The FDA also likes for a new drug to be tested against existing drugs on the market intended for the same purpose. Don't get me wrong. The FDA does not require these comparative tests. These are done only when they can be construed to make the new drug look better.

You might think that comparing two drugs would be quite straightforward. You probably don't read that many of these reports to the FDA.

The new drug is given to one group at what the manufacturer considers to be therapeutic dosages with a frequency they prefer. The comparison drug is commonly given far less frequently but at dosages five times or greater than has been its accepted usage. Those levels are considered to be either toxic or psychotoxic for many of the drugs.

Even with this advantage, the FDA usually forbids the manufacturer from advertising the new drug as more effective. Why? As I stated above, even with the biased studies the drugs did not demonstrate greater effectiveness than a placebo. Likewise, even with the little tricks the new drugs rarely, if ever, show themselves more effective than existing medications. None of the atypicals or SSRIs did.

The easiest way to find out how bad and ineffective a class of drugs is may surprise you. Just read what the manufacturer of the new drug says about the existing drug in these comparison studies.

Some of these assessments of the existing drugs are as critical as my own, only with much more detail and many more statistics. Manufacturers even provide the FDA with such critical comparisons to their own products; products that are about to lose, or have lost, their patent protection.

Another important factor in these tests is the duration. By far the most common length of time for conducting these tests is four to six weeks. While some side effects show up within a short span of time, that is not true for all, particularly many of the most serious ones. Some of the damage done by these drugs takes longer than six weeks to reach a critical point. Some take longer to exhibit themselves.

This industry leaves nothing to chance. If they prefer studies lasting six weeks, they have a reason. That reason is to minimize the appearance of serious side effects.

There is a question that crossed my mind not long after I began reviewing the studies. How can Agmina be sufficiently rational to volunteer for experimentation *(i.e.*, to take the drugs) but insufficiently rational to refuse treatment (*i.e.*, to refuse to take the drugs)? How convenient.

Another New Toy

Recently, there have been some studies of antidepressants using functional Magnetic Resonance Imaging (fMRI). These new studies have compared drug therapy with talk therapy and placebos. They have found that all three result in increased activity in the same areas of the brain. The increased activity they describe is regional cerebral blood flow.

You should be careful with studies employing fMRIs. Too many people, researchers included, jump to the conclusion that this increased activity somehow shows effectiveness. Listening to some researchers, and particularly as filtered through the media, one could easily get the impression that they have discovered the Holy Grail.

If there is a correlation between increased cerebral blood flow and beneficial results, no one has shown any proof or suggested any plausible mechanism. If the similarity of cerebral blood flow meant that they were accomplishing the same thing, why use the drug therapy? You know that the drugs have very serious side effects. You know that the talk therapy and placebos don't.

Even more fantastic claims for fMRIs seem to be made weekly, both in this field and others. They are now claimed to be excellent lie detectors. Just remember that every new drug, every new therapy, every new toy comes with claims bordering on the miraculous. These are very expensive toys and they need lots of reasons to use them to make them cost-effective.

I'm certain the real researchers will eventually find some advantage in fMRIs but you may be sure that the final list of usages will be considerably shorter and real miracles will return to being less than commonplace.

What actually happens is far more complex than simply increasing the flow of blood. While the results may appear or be similar on the macroscopic scale of regional cerebral blood flow, at the cellular level the mechanisms are entirely different. The multitude of other activities and processes don't show up on fMRIs. It is unlikely that increased blood flow is the most important or most interesting function taking place. Given those reservations, let me take you one step further into these tests.

Those receiving a placebo showed a rise from the beginning until they were told what they had been taking. Those receiving talk therapy also showed a rise from the beginning. Those taking a drug began with an initial dip before they started their rise. Since these medications are known to disrupt and damage the brain, while the sugar pills and talk therapy are not, it is a reasonable conjecture that the initial decrease represents that damage and/or disruption.

With all of the other data available, I maintain a fair degree of confidence that the subsequent rise can be blamed on the placebo effect or the real benefits of talk therapy. It would be expected that the action of the drug, after the initial damage was done, would be the same as the placebo, if the drug's effectiveness was due to the placebo effect. No surprise there. The odds of a drug emulating the placebo through its own devices are exceedingly long.

Little science is being done on the traditional tricyclics these days. As we know that the SSRIs are and perform basically as the older tricyclics, much of what we know about them is probably transferable to the older ones.

Good Pizza

MAOIs are little used these days because of all of the problems they present. Let me relate a personal experience with one of them. When it was prescribed for me, I was given a long list of dietary no-nos. Nothing with yeast was allowed. Bread is my favorite food. I often save my bread until last, almost as my dessert. Alcoholic beverages were verboten, especially beer. Every food I enjoyed seemed to be on that list.

It was probably 1982. My present wife and I were still in the dating stage. I was ensconced in a cottage on top of a mountain, overlooking a brow to an impressive valley, with the Smoky Mountains in the distance. I wasn't really enjoying the view. The flu had my immediate attention.

Snow was predicted for that evening and, the stereotypical single male, my larder was not well stocked. She called, expecting a live human being to pick up the phone, or at least an answering machine. Instead, she got a mumbling, sniffling vestige. She offered to make the trek up the mountain with some much needed rations.

Pizza. I was in such a state that even pizza looked good. I gulped down a slice. I started on a second slice. Uh-oh. Cheese. In my stupor and starving I had forgotten the list. A slice of pizza wasn't worth a brain aneurism but it may have been too late.

I called the poison control center. With my explanation of the situation the physician became quite obviously concerned. He asked if I were feeling dizzy. Did I have a headache? How much had I eaten? How long had it been? He was rifling through his books. He asked me to wait while he consulted a colleague.

He came back with a couple of more questions. Then another consultation. Then he asked me what brand of pizza. I told him it was a Godfather's.

He gave a huge sigh of relief. "You're okay. Godfather's doesn't use real cheese." I was relieved but still quite shaken by what had been seen as a close call. For some reason the question of yeast in the bread never came up during that phone call.

List in hand, I decided it was too easy to violate the dietetic strictures imposed by MAOIs. The possibility of a rebound be damned. I was not going to take any more of that class of medicine.

During this time the snow began to fall. The weatherman was predicting seven inches. Just in case Godfather's put yeast in the bread, or some other forbidden substance, I figured it was not best to be stuck on a mountain with a long, steep, gravel driveway.

I bundled up and trudged nearly half a mile uphill. She had been prescient enough to park at the entrance. Or, maybe it was just that she had never been fond of my driveway, even in the balmiest of weather.

It may be possible to abide by the restrictions but it is far too easy to forget. It would seem that most of the medical community has come to the same conclusion.

Unbreakable Chains

These people never give up. I'm certain that the remuneration involved is a consideration. It's also probable that many of them just can't break out of the intellectual cage. The old 'chemical imbalance' model is all they know. Despite all the evidence they believe it's the only answer . . . all it needs is just a little tweaking.

A popular alternative model is the reverse of what has been the true faith all these decades. Maybe we have too much serotonin or norepinephrine or something. Then, those expensive little pills increase that overabundance. How's that? Well, it seems that for this model to work the brain must have a way, a system for dealing with too much or too little of something.

The fact is it does have such a system - many of them. They were not permitted to exist under the old model. They provided answers for questions that were not allowed to be asked. The real problem is that they make alternatives to the standard model look rational.

But, as they finally cannot avoid the facts and are forced to give up on the old tried and false model, they seem incapable of straying too far (after all, they don't want to lose sales on the drugs they have and waste a lot of money on real research). However, they now need the very mechanisms that formerly were proscribed.

The new refrain is that Agmina have too much serotonin, or some monoamine and, if they give you one of those pills you used to take when they said you had a deficiency, you then will have even more of the very thing that is causing your problem. This will then cause one or more of these newly acknowledged systems to wake up and eliminate this new, putative excess.

This depends heavily on claiming that these systems refused to function as designed when the situation was only bad enough to traumatize you or bring on a suicide attempt or two. By taking the pill to make it even worse, for the same 3-4 weeks, it will still work almost as well as a placebo.

Why did not this newly-admitted system work to reduce the excess that was already there? Believe it or not, they have an explanation. It is kicked into action by an external agent.

Even though it's the same chemical compound, the externally boosted monoamine helps while the native excess of a monoamine without their help causes problems. See how prescient evolution was? It designed a mechanism millions of years ago in anticipation of Prozac.

Just as before, when the old model was true, the increase in the monoamine doesn't make you feel better, uh - oops, sorry; I mean worse. At least, it has no noticeable effect for the same 3-4 weeks. The new model says that the original excessive levels plus the new excessive levels of the monoamine cause down-regulation. This happens because either the number of receptors is reduced or the receptors are blocked or altered to become less sensitive.

Cynics might say that is a definition of brain damage but those of faith know that these supermen of science would never allow their products to cause harm.

Since it still takes 3-4 weeks for any effect, these prophets of the pill have estimated that, amazingly, down-regulation probably requires 3-4 weeks to work. It's a good thing that your sugar-insulin feedback system doesn't take that long.

I can't help but try to follow through on the rationale. The model says that the pill stimulates the brain to do the work. Now, if the mechanism in the brain down-regulates just enough to compensate for the new excessive level, we are right back where we started - minus the cost of the office visit and the medication.

If the brain down-regulates less than enough to compensate for the new excessive level, we are worse off than we were before. If the brain down-regulates enough to compensate for the new excessive level and more than enough for the old excessive level, we may have transformed a depressive into a manic.

Thankfully, these minions of mercy know just how much to prescribe. How they know that is apparently a trade secret. They admit that there is no existing test to determine the levels of monoamines in the brain, except postmortem. Maybe one size fits all. This could be the proof that we Agmina are all the same.

One last question now comes to mind. I am forced to suppose the prognosis that one must take these wonder drugs the rest of one's life hasn't changed just because the way we are told they work has changed. After all, if all Agmina begin taking drugs only for a few weeks instead of decades, the pharmaceutical industry will have to raise prices in Canada and every other country.

I guess that wasn't the final question. If one keeps on taking these pills that cause excessive levels of whatever monoamine, then aren't we either back where we started or continuing to kill off or shut off receptors until there are none left to do the work they are supposed to do? In the later case, how will those neurotransmitters facilitate communication in the brain without functioning receptors?

The only apparent answer is that one must stop short of killing off all the receptors. That means stopping the drugs at some point. Sorry, Mr. Lilly, *et al.*

Deficiency or excess - they don't know.

There are even more proposed models out there trying to save some shred of the discredited 'chemical imbalance' model but, believe it or not, they make even less sense. The lure of the old model has such a hold that many who understand the impossibility of it having any validity simply cannot break free.

Giving up on it would require learning something far less simplistic and, horror of horrors, not being able to manufacture facts on the fly, as required, to deny the unwanted realities. A real scientific model would not allow the nonsense that the 'chemical imbalance' model requires.

Too many seem unaware of the hold that the old model has on them. While these researchers are grasping at straws and all qualified researchers know that the old model is *kaput*, pharmaceutical companies, physicians, insurance companies, the FDA, APA, NIMH, NAMI and others keep pushing the pills on an enormous number of people in need of effective help and real care.

The researchers working on these variations are wasting much time and money that could be effectively spent on finding and implementing real solutions. Their ignorance allows the pharmaceutical companies to continue conning the public.

If not for those reasons I might feel compassion for them. I am inclined to feel sorry for those in situations beyond their resources, for people with limited intelligence, for . . . whoops, have I bought into some new stigma?

Recapping

Where are we? We have covered neuroleptics and their offspring, atypicals. We have covered tricyclics and their variation, SSRIs. We have briefly covered MAOIs. We know that none work to improve the psychiatric problems beyond a placebo effect, and not as well as placebos. All disrupt and/or damage the brain.

The theories that support their use do not withstand analysis. The theories are wrong. They are based on illogical assumptions. They are supported by falsified results, pseudoscience, reports commonly written by, or ghostwritten for, people without training as researchers and tons and tons of money. And we spend over $27 billion each year for this? We need therapies based on science, not marketing.

I have felt the helplessness that comes with the suicide of too many people I knew. I have shared the pain of many, many more friends and acquaintances. I am no longer defensive *vis-a-vis* these companies and their claims. It is time for them to defend their products and their actions. Fifty years of failure is enough. Fifty years of lies is enough.

If the products work, prove it. Tell us what depression is. Explain the mechanisms and states of it. Tell us what the products do to alter these states. Give us the lab results of the tests for monoamine levels (of live people). Absent that information, don't pretend to science. Don't pretend to help. Don't pretend to be honest. Don't pretend to have integrity. Don't pretend to have the scientific or moral standing to question any other models.

Humongous

For a period I was following the frequent fines levied against the drug companies; several hundred million dollars here, several hundred million dollars there. The largest fine to date was $875 million.

To you and me it sounds as though it would add up to real money but, given the immense profits after fines, these fines are just another cost of doing business. They have a negligible impact on the bottom line.

These are not simply large corporations as you might expect. They are special, very special. Ten pharmaceutical companies are listed among the Fortune 500. That's 500 of the largest companies in the United States. They may not be the top ten in size but, when it comes to profits, they are in a class by themselves.

In 2002 these ten companies had combined profits of $35.9 billion dollars. Okay, so they're big. The other 490 members of the Fortune 500 had combined profits of a bit more than $33.7 billion dollars. Ten companies had greater profits than 490 companies. There is a five-letter word that comes to mind. It begins with g-r-e-e and ends with the letter d.

Why are they fined? Sometimes it is for something simple, such as overcharging Medicare, Medicaid and insurance companies.

Sometimes it is for other illegal business practices. If you or I tried to rip off the government for just a few billion dollars, we would likely be in more trouble than just having to pay a fine representing a fraction of our take.

Killing for Money

Now we have the little Vioxx misunderstanding. The government estimates Vioxx caused or contributed to the deaths of 28,000 people over a certain period of time. That estimate covers only part of the time it was on the market.

First, we find that the company, the FDA and others had known of the problem since before it came on the market. We find that staff members at both the company and the FDA had pointed out the problem and been told to keep silent. Then the *New York Times* finds an internal memo dating back to 1996 delineating the problem.

1996 is four years before the government started counting the 28,000. They had the knowledge that it was deadly but kept everyone silent while raking in several billion dollars a year. How embarrassing.

It reminds me of a *New Yorker* cartoon. A group of executives sitting around a boardroom. The man at the head of the table says, "It's unethical. Does anyone have a problem with that?"

Still, even this partial count represents about ten times the number killed in the World Trade Center and Pentagon attacks of September 11, 2001. Interestingly, the number of people responsible for the decision to kill these victims was far fewer than the number of terrorists involved in the 9-11 attacks. They must be more elusive than much of *al-Qaeda*. We still haven't captured any of them.

They lie. They cheat. They steal. They kill. They do it for money. The chief executive officer of one of these firms made $150 million in one year. A chairman of the board's compensation was a mere $84 million that same year. None of the executives of these companies are on welfare. Their companies are (that's a whole 'nother story) but they're not.

None of the companies have been sentenced to death. None of the executives have served a day in prison. It might be too dangerous for them in prison. Over thirty percent of the prison population receives psychiatric services, which almost always means they are being treated with the products of these companies. Prisons are the largest repository of Agmina in this country.

If I were to call these people killers for hire, many people would say that was over the top. They would say I was being irresponsible. So, I won't say it. I'll just remind you that what you have read is factual, verified, much of it in the courts.

They have killed far more people for money than all of the Mafia's hit-men combined. Saying such things may upset some people. I hope so. There is more than sufficient reason to be upset with al-Pharma.

The trade association for the drug industry is called the Pharmaceutical Research and Manufacturers of America. They like to shorten it to PhRMA, pronounced pharma. Many writers and others refer to the industry as 'Big Pharma.' Admittedly, the industry is accurately termed 'Big' but I think my little twist better captures the essence, the spirit, the heart of this behemoth. So, al-Pharma it is.

The number of people we are told who were victims of Vioxx is appalling. We don't even have any estimates for the number Agmina dead as a result of these drugs. More people have taken them than Vioxx and for far longer periods of time.

Most studies have shown that suicides increase by sixty percent or so for people on various antidepressants. One study in Europe showed a 400% increase. Whatever the actual number, either larger or smaller than the Vioxx number, it is significant. Whatever the number, there has been no public outcry. Perhaps the terrorists would not be so reviled had they used drugs instead of planes or bought enough media and public servants.

Chapter 9

The Universe Weighs Three Pounds

If the brain were so simple we could understand it, we would be so simple we couldn't.

Lyall Watson

I am in awe of human beings. Sure, there are a number that I don't like. In a very real sense I am disappointed, distressed and disgusted by the failure of so many to take advantage of the potential and the abominable way so many treat their fellow human beings. We are capable of so much better.

Still, in a physical and biological sense, I am in awe. People look down on those with Turbiasis, Down's Syndrome and other limitations. I see it differently. Someone with so limited an intellectual capacity as to be unable to learn to read and write is still a marvel.

What brain power it takes to see, to feel, to taste, to hear, even to smell! Our understanding just of the physical senses is so primitive.

Even one as restricted as described above can speak, can communicate thoughts, desires, needs. That person can walk and maintain balance. That person can experience hunger and pain and make decisions to address those problems. That person can recognize family and friends; can perceive danger. That person will respond the same as you and me to being cut, to being kissed; being too long in a broiling sun or underdressed in a Winter storm.

Here we stand, without the ability to comprehend most of these simple matters in even the most superficial way. Do we have any appreciation of the marvel in front of us? No. For most people, a human being with so circumscribed an intellect is the object of ridicule, derision, contempt and scorn. How do we justify having so little regard for an organism so marvelous that neither you nor I will ever grasp a significant fraction of its beauty, its organization, its power, its complexity, its grandeur?

We even fail to exhibit due regard for fully functioning human beings seen as normal, particularly if they are in some way different; different in appearance, in culture or in dress. We find rejoicing over their misfortune or their destruction.

If the difference between the DNA of a human being and that of a chimpanzee is only 1.6 percent, how small is the difference between two people? More aptly, how much commonality is there between us? Most species of animals contain a greater diversity than do we. How we can show so little respect and regard for other creatures with whom we share so much in common is a mystery. Yes, I am very disappointed, distressed and disgusted with so many but still my awe is undiminished.

Going inside the brain one finds the same grey matter in everyone. Looking at the brain, whether as a whole or as a specimen under a microscope, you cannot tell me the color of that person, their gender, their religion, their age, their intelligence or most of their infirmities. Is that the brain of someone you love, someone you hate, someone you admire, someone you fear? The brain, even one of someone severely retarded, is more complex, more awe-inspiring than any other object of which we have experience.

Three pounds. That is a small fraction of one's total body weight but that little organ consumes twenty percent of one's energy. Under certain conditions it appropriates even more. Several organs may be vital but this one is what makes us who we are. It makes us human. It survives in a unique protective environment. It is surrounded and protected by the skull.

Apparently Nature decided no other organ deserved such security. There is a blood-brain barrier that also provides a measure of protection. This keeps most of the world at bay while allowing entrance to the essentials the brain requires for survival and functioning.

37 and Counting

I have seen the number of brain cells given as 100 million (100,000,000). I have also seen it claimed to be 100 billion (100,000,000,000). The second number is 1,000 times as large as the first. That is a fairly wide range but both numbers are far larger than we can truly grasp. I don't think anyone has actually counted.

If those numbers don't impress you, I'll try again. A single neuron is capable of having connections to up to 10 thousand (10,000) others. One estimate is that your brain has as many as 10 trillion (10,000,000,000,000) synaptic connections.

Many of you have heard of neurotransmitters - all three or four of them. You've probably heard of serotonin, dopamine, norepinephrine and maybe even epinephrine. The last two are known as noradrenalin and adrenalin in the British Isles, just in case you had heard of them and were confused. The reason most people think there are only three or four is because those are the only ones commonly mentioned.

In fact, there are more than 100 different neurotransmitters in your brain. This is further complicated by the fact that there is not a simple one-to-one match of neurotransmitter type with receptor type. As mentioned elsewhere, serotonin has 15 different known types of receptors. And, there are subtypes and sub-subtypes. You might find it helpful to think of these and the multitude of other compounds laying around in your brain as Tinker Toys. Most can be used in many different ways for many different purposes.

But, that is not all. There are neurohormones. There are neuropeptides. There are cytokines. There are neurokinins. There are glia. There are a host of goodies you likely have never heard of and unlikely to ever see mentioned again: brain-derived neurotrophic factor, substance-P, CREB (cyclic AMP-responsive element binding, a protein that turns on several genes to build new synapses involving the making of the memory of a shock) and such. Then there are the specialized parts: the thalamus, the hypothalamus, the pituitary, the amygdala, hippocampus and more.

It's kind of crowded in there. And we must not forget all the sugar in there. Glucose is the brain's food.

There is a good reason that this particular three pounds uses twenty percent of your energy. One helluva lot of activity is taking place up there. Hundreds of chemicals, each performing multiple tasks, dozens of specialized areas, billions of pieces and trillions of connections, require immense amounts of energy. All that activity means changes. The brain is constantly changing. The structure is ceaselessly being altered. The levels of these hundreds of chemicals are ever-changing.

Now, plug in the simpleminded concept of chemical imbalance. In such a complex organization of hundreds of compounds, performing thousands of functions, almost all in a perpetual state of ferment and flux, define chemical imbalance for us. Provide us the parameters of equilibrium. What a pitiful excuse for a scientific theory. What a pitiable band of experts are those who would believe it and use such nonsense as the foundation of treatment.

The profiteers of pharmaceutical fraud select one, two or three chemicals that provably have no direct bearing on Turbiasis. They admit that they don't know if or how they work, while insisting that they do. They acknowledge, as quietly as possible, that they can cause severe damage.

They conveniently forget to tell you that they have no way to tell you what your levels are. Based on this marvelous 'scientific' foundation, you are supposed to trust to them the very thing that makes you who you are, to accept their self-serving claims and to give them several billions of dollars each year. Let's ignore these charlatans for a while and concentrate on facts and logic.

Don't Jump

I hope to cover enough of the parts and workings of the brain to help you understand, if not the brain itself, at least the foundations of the new model of Turbiasis. Be aware that it is possible, indeed probable, that you will be spurred by a comment here or there on a relationship of chemicals, parts or processes to jump towards what appears to be an obvious logical extension. This is sometimes so seductive that even real researchers often go astray.

I would not hazard a guess as to how many papers I've seen that have been based on ill-advised, precipitous leaps. They see that the solution was so easy that others will see the same connection and beat them to it. They usually rush to contact a reporter, to ensure they get the credit. One academic paper, one newspaper article, sometimes even a short little flurry of articles, fifteen minutes of fame, and then embarrassment. I will try to remember, when a good example presents itself, to point out such a pitfall.

It appears the time has come to get down to the knee-bone-connected-to-the-neck-bone part, the nitty-gritty, the nuts and bolts. Parts of this chapter may seem daunting to a layman.

Don't worry if the glut of new words or the specific connections, parts and processes fail to stick in your mind with the insistence of your favorite commercial jingle. For the general reader, just try to get some feel for what goes on, its importance and its implications. The rest will be, for the most part, in familiar territory.

The public uses the word stress to cover both the external events and elements that may be the cause and the reactions of the body and brain to those stimuli. Neuroscientists have separated the two. The former, the stimuli, remain stresses. The reaction is termed allostasis. The researchers have found that the body is always prepared and constantly adjusting, constantly trying to maintain a state of equilibrium. An environmental stress is seen to represent a threat and the brain and body react to protect themselves, you. This dynamic operation to protect you and return the systems to a state of equilibrium is allostasis.

If you are subjected to stresses too frequently, the brain and body may have trouble answering the call. The system may suffer damage. Parts may work erratically or cease to work. When allostasis cannot be maintained, you have probably thought of it as being stressed out. Now you can call it an allostatic load, as the professionals do.

The Axis

Allostasis is centered around three parts of the brain and body. These are the hypothalamus (residing in the brain), pituitary gland (also residing in the brain) and the adrenal glands (sitting atop the kidneys, hopefully not in the brain). This becomes the hypothalamic-pituitary-adrenal axis, the HPA axis for convenience. The actions of the HPA axis are far-reaching. The neuroscientists usually refrain from calling this the allostatic system. They have their reasons.

The body and brain have a host of systems. The HPA axis, in various situations, may need to call one or more of these systems into action. I appreciate their reasons for not calling it a system but consider it more convenient to call it and think of it in terms of a system.

Because the HPA axis relies so heavily on other components and systems, the scientists are correct in not referring to it as a separate system but I conceive of the allostatic system as the super-system. It acts upon and is acted upon by all the other systems. Just think of the HPA axis as the director of this super-system.

So complex a system is liable to problems. There are numerous potential points of disruption or failure. As noted, the levels and types of stress that can impinge upon the system are varied and growing. Putting excessive stress on any system is a recipe for trouble.

The reader is surely familiar with the idea that some people are more susceptible than others to cancer or other diseases. One person may smoke for fifty years and die of kidney failure while another succumbs to lung cancer in a span of less than five years.

We might speak of this as a lower threshold, a greater sensitivity or in some other way. The complex nature of our body and brain allow for the cause in one person to be a lower threshold, while in another the cause may be a greater sensitivity or for one of the other postulated reasons.

A system with so many elements, involved in so many critical functions, with a plethora of increasing pressures on many of its constituent parts, is likely to have more than one way of failing to work as intended.

Some people have, as some do with cancer, a sensitivity or lower threshold to stress. It may be the result of a sensitivity to adrenalin, to cortisol or some other agent. It may be the result of an abnormal level of production of one of these compounds.

There could be a failure of one of the several feedback mechanisms. There could be a component part of the system that does not function normally. Any of these problems could be, and more than likely are, the result of an abnormal expression or repression of one or more genes. This is where the factor of heredity comes into play.

I stated that it is more than likely that the problem is one of genetics. The prominence of heredity has been recognized for centuries. The potential for heredity to play a role in the allostatic system is certain. There are, in fact, a multitude of points in this system where a faulty gene expression, or repression, can have an effect.

People both with Turbiasis and people free of it have been shown to have above normal, below normal and normal levels of the various monoamines. No heredity association or rational proposal for a genetic explanation for abnormal monoamine levels exists. A 'chemical imbalance' model finds no support here.

Gene expression is not the only method for damaging or disrupting the system. This is where stress enters the picture. An element of the allostatic system that is not capable of functioning normally may be induced to function abnormally when called on by the system. I say may because there are various types of stressors and a particular element of the system may not be called into play for some of these.

As noted elsewhere, while stress may appear as a sabertooth tiger, it also may appear as a virus, a hubritic boss, an irate customer, a traffic jam, a paper cut, etc. The response of the system to these will be different, involving different parts of the system. This not only allows for differentiation, it requires it.

While genetics can explain the bulk of the cases of Turbiasis, it doesn't address them all. Every component of the allostatic system is subject to abuse, dysfunction and failure.

For those with normal systems, stress will bring the system into play but equilibrium usually will return under the aegis of the allostatic system, as is to be expected. However strong and resilient a normal system may be, it does have its limits.

A sufficient level of stress, either in one instance or by accumulation over a period of time, can cause the system to function abnormally. The less mature or more aged the brain, the more vulnerable to stress.

Children are particularly susceptible to permanent damage from excessive stress. Given enough stress of the proper kind, everyone is at risk of failure of some part or parts of the system. If the dysfunction happens to certain parts of the system, acutely enough, Turbiasis can result.

Let me emphasize the significance of the last paragraph. Anyone can suffer from Turbiasis. Everyone is susceptible. No one is immune.

The odds are overwhelming that when this occurs to a person with a normal allostatic system it will express itself as a depression. The probability is that the normal system has sufficient strength and resilience to recover, to return to normal functioning. This is known as situational depression.

Previously, many considered situational depression to be different than chronic depression to a greater extent. The precipitant cause is the same and the mechanism is the same. The differences are the level of stress needed to initiate it and the prognosis. The prognosis for situational depression is good. The normal duration will usually fall within a range of six weeks to six months.

Saying the prognosis is good, I mean to apply that to the duration only. Depression is depression. The descriptives of chronic and situational tell you nothing of the severity or the reaction of the individual. Different personalities in differing circumstances will respond differently. Either form of depression can end in suicide or attempts.

One last thought before leaving this. Even though recovery is highly likely, there is no guarantee that permanent damage will not result. If it does, the form of depression becomes chronic. For anyone disposed to buy into the stigma, to mistreat, look down on or ridicule Agmina, it would be wise to remember that the future may place you among us. It would behoove every presently normal person not to indulge in or encourage statements or actions that would reinforce the stigma.

I jumped a bit ahead of myself here but it seemed unavoidable or at least not too worrisome a situation nor worth trying to straighten it all out for the purists, who likely gave up long ago. No harm.

Chapter 10

Wake Up

You will soon break the bow if you keep it always stretched.
Phaedrus

What is stress? We are all very familiar with stress. We experience it daily. We talk about it. So, what more is there to know? I would like to take you on a short trip. I would like to take you through a typical day.

The alarm fails to go off this morning. You're late. Stress. You forgot to buy new razor blades and in your hurry you nick yourself several times. Stress. You run out to bring in the newspaper and are confronted by a large, growling, feral dog. Stress. The little wife yells at you, reminding you, as though it were really necessary, that you are late. Stress. You hop in the car. The starter grinds away for several seconds before the engine turns over. Just a little more stress.

You get on the freeway and come to a complete stop. This day's traffic is a bit worse than usual, and you are running late. Stress. With too much frequency, idiots in other cars keep you on edge by forcing their way into the seven and a half inches between your front bumper and the rear bumper of the car in front of you. Stress. You finally get an open stretch and use the opportunity to catch up. Blue lights and a siren. Stress.

Finally, you arrive at work. The boss sees you trying to sneak in and gives you a snarl. Stress. Later, he drops an important project on your desk that is already overdue. Stress. The Coke machine takes your money; the copy machine gets jammed; the monitor on your computer goes to the famous blue screen. Just a little more stress. You get fired. Someone in Sri Lanka will do your job for fifty-seven cents a day. Stress. You arrive home to the security and comfort of your hearth, to the support of your family. Your wife yells at you for losing your job, as though that was necessary. Stress.

I think there is general agreement that each and every one of the incidences described above would qualify as stressful to a greater or lesser degree. But there were, or could have been, other things going on that day that we might have not known to be stressing us or might have known about but categorized as simply frustrating or inconvenient.

You get out of bed that morning. That brings on stress. Your body must transition from a resting state to one of activity. The heart rate increases. The blood pressure rises. Your body must increase the supply of oxygen to your muscles. That is stress. You didn't have time to eat breakfast. Your brain realizes that you need to replenish your energy supplies. You need food. Pangs of hunger strike you. That is stress.

You get in your car on a crisp, cool morning and the heater in the car takes some time before putting out heat. You're cold. That activates the stress system. You don't know it but you just picked up a virus. Your stress system has to activate the immune system. You get to work and notice that your socks don't match. Is that merely frustrating or inconvenient? Maybe, but it's also stressful. You give yourself a paper cut. Again, the immune system needs to kick into gear.

After such a day, your dinner may not sit well. You may experience diarrhea or vomiting. Not only is that stressful but perhaps it is your body's stress system reacting to earlier stresses. You finally get to bed. You think you have a brief respite from stress. You snore. Once again, stress comes into play. Your heart and other organs and system must work harder.

Just another typical day. You may be forgiven, except by your loving spouse, for being a bit touchy, a bit grouchy, just a little on edge. You don't feel well, and why not? Stress has brought all your major organs and some of your systems into play on an almost constant basis. Your body put in a great deal of overtime. Your resources were strained, some perhaps were damaged.

Stress is good. From the reams of studies, discussions and reports devoted to stress, one easily gets the impression that stress is an unalloyed evil. Stress is good and bad. It's just that there are many kinds of stress. It makes no more sense to express a singular judgment on stress as either good or bad than it does to aver that all plants are edible or that all plants are poisonous.

Given the constant drumbeat telling of the harm and dangers of stress, how can it be a beneficial factor? Well, it's only beneficial if you wish to live.

Stress is absolutely necessary to the survival of any organism. Without stress, you die. There are other aspects of stress which have their use but that one alone should be adequate for most people.

Looking at the stresses mentioned above, we know that not everyone of those will cause problems for everyone. We do, however, need to be aware of the total effect. Several of those may come into play on top of either a major stressful event or as the straw that finally causes the camel his back problem. Another apt analogy may be the constant dripping of a faucet.

Just to be sure and touch all bases, stress can, on some occasions, depending on type and degree, have an essentially neutral result as well. Nothing I have said to this point concerning stress is meant to minimize the very real threat that stress represents. That threat is to everyone but is, or should be, of particular interest to those with a stake in Turbiasis.

Stress is an evolutionary mechanism developed to help protect human beings. Actually, it was developed for our predecessors. We just inherited and modified it. It provides the body with a greater amount of short-term strength and energy. This enables a person to be more powerful in a fight or to have greater speed and stamina in flight. For an extended period of man's existence, this had been a boon. As matters have developed, however, there is less and less need for some of these modes of self-protection.

The reduced need does not translate into a reduction of stress, though. The pace of modern life brings a multitude of situations and factors that induce stress.

When we are stressed, for whatever reason, adrenalin and cortisol are sent coursing throughout our system. Every cell of our body is affected. Our entire body reacts. Our heartbeat speeds up in order to deliver more blood everywhere. This is the body's method for increasing the level of oxygen available. Increased oxygen feeds the muscles, giving greater potential power and endurance. It also sends white blood cells scurrying throughout the body to deal with cuts, infections, *etc.*

The immune system will be called upon in case we are wounded but, if it is pushed too far, it is impaired, it opens the individual to any number of other maladies. Many other aspects of the body, various organs and operations, are similarly affected. All of this is intended to benefit us for the short-term.

The problem is that, while enhancing the body's ability to protect itself, cortisol stretches the body's limits, at both the system and cellular level. This benefactor exacts a price. It does some damage to the recipient. It destroys cells. It weakens the bones. It damages organs.

Among the cells destroyed are those in the brain. It does this to a minor extent even when it is used for the intended purpose. It is capable of doing more damage to other areas when the muscles and other systems related to fight or flight fail to use the augmented capabilities.

Repeated stress brings additional opportunities to inflict additional damage to the brain, as well as other areas. Each episode results in further damage to the body and brain.

When?

In general terms, stress is the precipitating factor for psychotic episodes. Late adolescence is a most common time for Turbiasis to first rear its ugly head in a fashion that is unquestionably apparent. Why should this be? Is there some sort of internal clock or timing mechanism associated with Turbiasis? Not really. It just happens to be a time that, in our society, puts upon young people a great deal of stress.

Kids have been cocooned in a special, artificial atmosphere through secondary school. It is all they know but it is a haven which they must leave, and to which they will never return. In all those years they have been scheduled and guided through the educational system.

Classes are usually consecutive and daily. They know where to be, where to proceed to that next 50- or 55-minute block of time. Failure to be where their schedule designates when the schedule dictates will be noted by the system. The system will work to rectify such minor aberrations. Their responsibility is limited to being where they are supposed to be at the proper time and accomplishing the tasks selected for them.

Then comes the pomp and circumstance. At long last, for the first time in their memory, they have a taste of freedom, a taste of adulthood. As we all later learn, these are not unmixed states. They come to us with requirements of responsibility, obligation, accountability and the need to make consequential choices.

Those minor matters are not evident to these fledglings at first blush. They just revel in their newfound situation. The reality soon breaks through this fragile veneer of euphoria.

For the most part, these newly minted adults go in one of two directions: college or the work force. Both of these courses represent a significant change from their formative experiences.

The collegiate setting and context is considerably different than one's previous educational experience. Your classes are likely to be non-consecutive. Some are likely to be hour sessions on Monday, Wednesday and Friday. Others will be an hour and a half on Tuesday and Thursday.

You have the responsibility of adjusting everything else in your schedule around those classes. Now it's totally up to you.

No one else will shepherd you around. No one in all this large, busy community, no one in this vast new universe in which you find yourself seems to even have any concern for whether or not you show up for your classes. You're not in 'Kansas' anymore.

It's possible to drift lazily through that first semester completely oblivious to the consequences. It's possible to enjoy the distractions of this newfound freedom to the detriment of the reason you or your parents are going into debt. It's possible to wander through this new world in such a state for only a limited period.

The time comes all too quickly when the real world will no longer be denied. It usually comes in the form of grades, just a little piece of paper recording your failure to measure up to the standards of this new world. With this comes a confrontation with some factotum from the college. Then there is the parents' displeasure, reproach and censure. Here we have a perfect description, if not the definitive definition, of stress.

This is, of course, not the only available path to stress that one can find in college. There are the unfamiliar surroundings. There is the absence of family and friends. One may realize at this time the important roles played by the people who have made up one's support system. The proximate cause could be any one of these or other factors, or some combination but the result is still stress.

A recent study showed one-third of college students reporting some symptoms of Turbiasis. One major university said that fifteen percent of the student body were receiving psychiatric services from the school. Given the reluctance of many to seek services or admit, even to themselves their need for help, such figures are only indicative, not a precise measure of the need.

Another factor to consider is the devalued state of a high-school education. The economy puts little value on such a diploma.

This has driven more people to college. Many enroll in college because they feel the need, not because they would ordinarily choose to attend. Many of these are academically unprepared or unsuited. Finding oneself in this position can understandably lead to increased stress.

Is it really necessary to list the differences between being a high school student and a brand new, full-fledged member of the workforce? Let's just say that the changes are many and drastic. The frustrations, the impositions and the challenges are seemingly endless.

The various types of stress that can accompany either of these new environments offer one an extensive menu from which to choose.

Another potential factor bringing stress to those going into the workforce is that of lost opportunities. One may enter the marketplace not from a positive desire or personal choice but due to circumstances, economic or otherwise, that frustrate a desire for the alternative of furthering one's education. Frustration over such matters as this, among many, many other causes, represents a large portion of the roots of stress.

Stress may also be induced by various insults to the body, including, but not limited to the brain. Illnesses, toxins, pollution, even medications, all can precipitate a release, indeed, even a massive surge of chemicals from the array available. It is impossible to avoid all stress but we must learn to understand its role, recognize it and deal with it.

Stress may come relatively quickly or otherwise. It may result from a sudden loss of a family member or any number of other events which bring about an acute trauma. It may also build up over a period of years. In this last situation, one takes on, at some point, what is described as the straw that broke the dromedary's back.

As variegated as are both the causes and manifestations of stress, we need also to recognize the various ways with which people deal with it. Certain people may, in essence, ignore particular pressures or situations that might qualify as stressful to others. Sometimes it is possible to minimize or eliminate the stress reaction, or its cause. Then again, one may learn to deal with stress in a way that negates some of its adverse effects.

People are different. A type of stress that is harmful to one person may have little or no apparent effect on someone else. That particular stress may even be useful. As remarked upon above, college is often so stressful for many as to precipitate psychotic episodes. My own experience is quite the opposite.

During periods when I was otherwise incapacitated and unable to obtain or maintain employment, I knew that I could return to the Groves of Academe. I thrived in an academic environment. School became a comfortable, protective retreat, a haven.

This reinforces the point that one cannot lump all Agmina into a single, undifferentiated mass. Turbiasis does not turn its prey into an army of identical clones. It very well may alter one's personality but it does not deprive one of his or her individuality.

A Success Story

A few years ago I was working on a federal demonstration grant from the National Institute of Mental Health. The purpose was to organize self-help groups in rural areas statewide. I had an office in a small, centrally located town. The bulk of my time was spent away from that office, so I needed a point of contact.

From the group I had organized in that town, I selected a young woman who had the time available to answer my phone calls. In her late twenties, she was the single parent of a 12-year old son. The plan was to call her when I was ready to leave the office and forward my calls to her home.

I met her at the local Shoney's for coffee. She bought into the stigma. She had no self-confidence whatever. She wanted to help but felt she could not handle the assignment. It took nearly three hours to convince her that she was fully capable. The waitress wasn't too happy that we were taking up one of her tables for such an extended period for the price of coffee for two. She was mollified when I left a tip that was somewhat more than is customary for two coffees.

Back to the story. This young lady desperately wanted to better herself. She wanted to be an occupational therapist. She had enrolled in the local state technical college five times. Never was she able to last more than three weeks. The stress did her in each time.

Over those endless refills I related some of the struggles and successes I had experienced. She could identify with some of those struggles. She saw that Turbiasis was not necessarily a dead end. She had met someone who had Turbiasis but had also managed an occasional success. She learned that it was not impossible.

Reluctantly, she agreed to try to handle my calls. The young lady did an excellent job of getting my messages to me. A bit more than a year later, it turned out that she had a surprise announcement for me. Without telling me, she had once again enrolled in school. She had very successfully completed the first year of her training to be an occupational therapist. Was I really that good of a counselor? No. As a peer, as one who shared some of her problems, I had a credibility with her that a psychiatrist, psychologist or social worker could not match.

As one who could provide concrete proof that success is possible for Agmina, my example shattered the stereotype for her. Someone cared. Someone shared. Someone needed her. Someone trusted her. It helped her understand that the stigma was not founded on facts. Our long, caffeine-sotted session was only the spark. It gave her hope. It was a challenge for her as she dealt time and again with the doubts and self-abnegation she had experienced in all of those previous attempts. A different perspective had made it easier for her to deal with the stress inherent in the situation for her.

Her life was changed, not by a prescription, not by the paid ministrations of someone with meaningless credentials, not by electrical shock.

Her life was changed by someone caring enough to establish rapport with her, by giving her concrete proof that there was hope, by giving her an opportunity.

Late in Coming

It is little recognized that many people with Turbiasis will never experience any noticeable symptoms and will never realize they have the disease. These people will pass on the genes, however.

How can they have the illness but not know? As stated earlier, it takes stress to bring about a psychotic episode or other problems of a lesser degree.

It may be that the person experiences either an insufficient level of stress or fails to encounter the particular kind of stresses that he or she has not the ability to successfully deal with.

While attending a conference at the University of California at Berkeley, I met a lady with symptoms somewhat similar to, and a diagnosis the same as, my own. She was in her mid-sixties.

As with others, her first awareness that she had Turbiasis was the instance of her first psychotic episode. That first episode was fairly recent; just a couple of years previous to our meeting. Why was the disease so late in manifesting itself in her?

The lady was a retired schoolteacher. With no spouse or children of her own, her career had been her life. She had been important. She had been important because she was needed. Then, of a sudden, she saw herself as no longer needed.

Whether the realization of this was, initially, conscious or unconscious, it represented an insult to her psyche. It precipitated stress.

Even though it came at a relatively late period in life, stress finally delivered her first psychotic episode. With that occurrence came the realization that she was a member of the Agmina.

When the appropriate level and kind of stress appears to one with that dormant disease, it makes itself known. A person reading this book may know that they have Turbiasis but no one reading this book is guaranteed that they are free of it.

Everywhere You Look

Just concentrate on the fact that more than one in five have the illness. Make a habit of looking around you. Are there five or more in your family? How many people are there in your workplace? Estimate the number of people in the restaurant, or supermarket, or church, or standing in line at the post office. Divide by five.

Since it is a bit greater than twenty percent, if there is a sizeable number in the vicinity, you might need to add a little to the resulting figure. Furthermore, even those without a genetic predisposition can join our special little group, given sufficient stress.

Any time you see someone with Turbiasis being abused, belittled or otherwise mistreated, perhaps you should remember that you very well could suffer the same. If you wish to be treated more humanely, if and when you are stricken, it is incumbent that you begin working towards that end immediately.

Discover how it feels to be denied any credibility. Look seriously into the common affronts to one's dignity. Study the side effects of the medications.

Watch for ways that you and others bring unnecessary stress upon Agmina, individually and collectively. Consider if you want to be treated as a sentient and sensitive human being or as an object of mindless humor and derision, as something less than fully human.

Dr. Fred Frese, who lives with schizophrenia, has created a little card for himself and others to hand out in appropriate circumstances. It says:

> I need to tell you that I am a person suffering from a mental disorder. When I am berated, belittled, insulted or otherwise treated in an oppressive manner, I tend to become emotionally ill. Could I ask that you restate your concern in a manner that does not tend to disable me? Thank you for your consideration.

When it involves Turbiasis, people do seem to need to be reminded that one with an illness should be treated with consideration.

Okay, so maybe it won't be you. It might only be a spouse, a sibling or one of your children. Does that make you less concerned?

Turbiasis is so devastating and has such pervasive effects on the individual that it greatly involves and affects those close to the person. It destroys marriages. It alienates parents and children.

Stress is the initiating and aggravating factor. It is also a common result for both the Agmina and those around them. Every credible estimate I have seen shows stress-related illnesses as accounting for half or more of the visits to primary care physicians. Reading lists of these illnesses almost leaves you wondering if there are any not involving stress.

Those estimates need to be revised upwards, however. They did not include Turbiasis. The researchers in the field of allostasis seem confident that autoimmune diseases are caused by stress. We could easily be talking about two-thirds or three-quarters of these visits being caused by stress.

Perhaps just a partial list of diseases that are stress related would be in order here.

Anorexia nervosa
Atherosclerosis
Rheumatoid arthritis
Hyperthyroidism
Hypothyroidism
Cushing's syndrome
Chronic fatigue syndrome
Fibromyalgia
Eczema
Ulcers
Bulimia
Allergies
Heart Attack
Diabetes
Stroke
Influenza
Colitis
Asthma
Colds
Infections

Even in such a partial list the range in the types of disorders is notable. The reason is clear. As we saw in the previous chapter, stress, through the HPA axis, has both direct and indirect effects on every system in the body. Add all of those autoimmune disorders and Turbiasis to the above and you have a good impression of the scope of the problem of stress.

Actually, we could add a few more complaints to the above list. They are not diseases. Rather, they are symptoms. Problems with sleep, sex drive, appetite and some others are not symptoms of depression, as we are generally told. They are symptoms of stress.

In fact, depression itself might be construed as a symptom of stress. But, as with those on the list above, depression is so serious as to be classified as an illness or disease, rather than as merely a symptom, regardless of its cause. Although manic-depression and schizophrenia are more involved than depression, stress plays a major role in them as well.

Can you imagine the savings in money, resources and misery society would experience were we to reduce the effects of stress by even marginal amounts? We could refurbish our nation's infrastructure. We could improve our educational system. We could attack the myriad social ills that plague us.

Let's begin to dip our toes into the allostatic system. The HPA axis, as stated earlier, acts as the control center for the other systems. As good a place to begin as any would be the autonomic nervous system.

It has three separate components. The sympathetic nervous system turns on the power. The visceral afferent system is a network of nerves from the organs to the brain through which the brain can pick up messages from the various parts of the body. The parasympathetic nervous system turns off the power or, we might say, restores the status quo.

I speak of turning power on and off. Just what do I mean? Turn what on and off? Well, the sympathetic nervous system increases pulse and blood pressure. The parasympathetic nervous system decreases them. Is that all? No. Add in the lungs, stomach, liver, pancreas, kidneys, intestines, rectum, bladder, sexual organs and more.

Sometimes one part acts on one or more organs. Sometimes the other one is active. Sometimes both are active. The brain is receiving signals as to what is taking place. The brain responds. The HPA axis is actively involved.

I have just quickly skimmed over one of the systems that is involved. I provided almost no detail and, already, you cannot miss the hints of complexity.

The immune system. The cholinergic system. And the peripheral nervous system. The cardiovascular system. The limbic system. The homeostasis systems. The endocrine system. The reproductive system. The portal-hypophysial capillary system. The mesocortical system. The nigrostriatal system. We could go on all day.

In regurgitating this partial list of systems it occurred to me that a word of caution might be in order. Don't think of these divisions in too precise a set of terms.

One research team works on one problem and defines the physical scope of its study as a system. Another team does the same with a different problem. The criteria for describing, defining and classifying a system are fluid, perhaps *ad hoc*. When speaking of one system, we may be including parts or the entirety of one or more other systems.

We know that stress damages areas of the brain that control mood. In other words, stress causes Turbiasis. We also know that stress causes damage to organs and systems that result in heart disease, diabetes, asthma and a host of other problems. The proof is there and the connection of stress to Turbiasis and stress to all of those other, somatic problems is absolutely straightforward.

Although the former connection is there in the literature for all to see, it hasn't been recognized, or there would be no need for a major part of this book. Given that it is, and has been, there for a period covering all of the careers of most researchers, their difficulty in seeing it is amazing.

Recent interviews with some researchers have elicited a strange new perception. They see the damage to the various organs involved with the somatic problems. They know that they can be caused by stress. They see this damage far more frequently in people with Turbiasis than they do in the general population. They postulate that Turbiasis is causing the damage.

That is evidence that the propounding and expounding of the stress-damage model of Turbiasis is necessary. Stress causes both the Turbiasis and the problems that exhibit themselves as physical ailments. The inability of the research community to see what is so plain is attributable to the intellectual fog and fictional science created by the drug makers with the marketing of the 'chemical imbalance' model.

Chapter 11

Say What?

> *We all agree that your theory is crazy, but is it crazy enough?*
> Niels Bohr

> *The greatest challenge to any thinker is stating the problem in a way that will allow a solution.*
> Bertrand Russell

The answer is simple, straightforward and has been in front of us for a very long time. I say the answer is simple. In a sense it is. When we are dealing with the brain, however, we will ever encounter complexity. The answer is both simple and complex.

It is not in dispute that stress is a contributing factor, an exacerbating factor in the appearance of psychotic episodes. There is evidence that a role for stress was recognized by the ancient Greeks and, before them, the Egyptians. It now seems such a small step to see stress as the very causative factor of Turbiasis itself.

If you are going down a dead end road in the wrong direction and being constantly told by the high priests that you have arrived at the destination, it's understandable that there might be a delay in getting to where you really need to go. The 'chemical imbalance' theory, the drug companies and the medical community have impeded the journey.

The most common way of acquiring Turbiasis is via heredity. How? You may have a genetic predisposition to produce too much cortisol. You may have a genetic predisposition of lower tolerance for cortisol. You may have a greater sensitivity to cortisol. The feedback mechanism for turning off the production of cortisol may malfunction. All of these are inheritable.

Just with the single question of cortisol we find there are several potential problems that could lead to Turbiasis. Those mentioned above are not the only ones. Neither is a problem directly related to cortisol the only way we have of developing the disease.

You can see by any listing of the various and diverse types of symptoms involved that it is not as simple as pointing at a solitary factor. One may inherit one, two or all of the necessary anomalies necessary to experience Turbiasis. One may inherit less than all of the necessary anomalies and never experience it. One may inherit less than all of the necessary anomalies and acquire the other(s) by some damage caused by stress.

People who think they do not have Turbiasis may be right. However, they may be short only one or two of those specific factors needed. They may have none of the factors. Still, neither of these groups are guaranteed to remain free of the disorder. The allostatic system is too pervasive and stress too common to think that anyone is exempt. While no one is exempt, genetics gives some people a head start.

The number of parts of the brain and body (remember the adrenal gland), the number of feedback mechanisms, the number of chemicals, the number of functions each of several parts and chemicals play and the complex interplay of all of these provide an untold number of ways something could go wrong. This multitude of possible problems will exhibit themselves as a variety of combinations of symptoms. There is no panacea. One pill is not the answer. Three classes of pills are not the answer.

Let me at this point qualify my assertion that stress is the cause of Turbiasis. Television personality Jane Pauley recently made public her own bout with manic-depression. She contends that it was the result of taking a medication for hives. I have no knowledge of the evidence upon which her physician reached this conclusion but find it a very distinct possibility.

Looking into the biology and physiology of the brain, there definitely are points of susceptibility to pharmacological insults. Of all those possible locations for disruption of the super system, the allostatic system, mentioned in the previous chapter, some are undoubtedly susceptible to a drug.

I have not pursued a determination of which pharmacological agents might have the potential to induce Turbiasis but agree that there likely are several. My guess is that corticosteroids would be at or near the top of any such list.

In essentially the same manner as medication can activate Turbiasis, some viruses also appear to have the capacity to do so. Which ones? That is not presently known.

There is no allowance in the 'chemical imbalance' model for an explanation of how either a medication or a virus could be the cause of Turbiasis. There is a place for these in the stress-damage model.

Stress activates the allostatic system, where all the fun begins. A virus will activate the allostatic system. Why? Because to the allostatic system it represents a threat, a stress factor.

Some medications also bring it into play. Either can be a factor but we must bow to and acknowledge the complexities of both the brain and the disease. We can say with great certainty that one of these may be a factor but unlikely to be sufficient in and of itself. In other words, they commonly will need help. Multiple factors would usually be needed to develop Turbiasis. The fact that Turbiasis exhibits itself with multiple symptoms makes it unlikely that a single, discrete factor can account for all of them.

In Ms. Pauley's case it is likely that other factors were in place and the stress represented by that particular medication, or the virus itself, acted upon the part of her allostatic system that was the necessary final component required for the expression of Turbiasis. That explains why not everyone taking that medication experiences Turbiasis.

If these are stresses, then they fall wholly within the simply stated maxim above that stress is the cause of Turbiasis. If you were to separate them out as being a bit different than say, hereditary factors, you could have some grounds for doing so but the delineation might not have all the clarity and specificity you might wish.

At this point we cannot trace each path and list each organ and each chemical or give numeric values to the degrees of normal functioning of the various parts. The possible variations are unknowable at present. How much commonality and/or difference there is between the involved parts and pathways brought into play by different stimuli is no more than conjecture today.

I know that the picky we shall always have with us. They will say that I have admitted to several causes: genetic, pharmacological, viral, *et al*. Someone always then asks what percentage of Turbiasis is caused by each. This is a case of *caveat lector*.

I have been tempted to guesstimate that genetics cover at least eighty-five percent. Why? I don't know. It's the result of trying to be responsive to the question without getting bogged down in a long and detailed exposition, simply to admit that it is presently unknowable.

It represents no more nor less than what I feel is a quite reasonable approximation. My feelings, expressed as a guess, should not be taken to the bank or engraved in stone.

So when, as we go along, I write that Turbiasis is caused by stress, please understand that I am not ignoring the superficially apparent variations. Just remember, stress can come to us in a multitude of flavors.

Stress as the causal factor answers lots of questions. It offers a perspective that allows for questions that can't emerge from the simplistic 'chemical imbalance' theory. It stimulates us to look to new areas for consideration that have potential for advancing our knowledge, developing new therapies and getting past the inanities of the stigma.

The percentage of people with Turbiasis is growing faster than the general population. There is growth of the illness across the age spectrum: in adolescence, young adulthood, middle age and my group, the decrepit and senile. The first psychotic episode was most likely to occur in the late teens or early twenties. That has been creeping downward. Why? Just consider the changes in our society. You would be hard-pressed to find anyone to disagree that our society has become more stressful. Change has been with us for quite some time but the pace has picked up and continues to do so.

The economy has done its part. Job security is apt soon to be found only in history books. Outsourcing is rarely celebrated outside of executive suites, corporate boardrooms and the State of India. McDonald's and Burger King have made heroic efforts to fill the breech but serving hamburgers to each other doesn't strike me as the strongest foundation upon which to build an economy. If gas prices keep going up, we may even find ourselves visiting the drive-thru windows on bicycles.

The correlation of increased stress and growth in the numbers of people afflicted with Turbiasis is more than suggestive. It answers questions that were not and could not be entertained before. The mechanism to link the two is straightforward and logical. The pieces of the puzzle quite easily start falling into place.

A great number of would-be super parents are pushing themselves and their children to an extent that is both unwise and unhealthy. Soccer moms did not become such a popular political codeword in the absence of such or for a relatively small number. Karate, dance, Little League, cheerleading, music, after-school tutoring and home schooling represent a heavy load. Perhaps it would be advisable to drop one or two.

My mother's obsession to fulfil her thwarted ambitions through her offspring seemingly has become a national pastime. While my mother's efforts were fueled by her personal psychoses, the strength of the national trend may be said to have reached the point of being a societal one. Few of these obsessed parents will be any more successful than mine in creating a combination world-class athlete/genius. Many will, however, push their children to the point of neurosis, psychosis, suicide, the next Columbine or some other unintended situation or state.

It's not just the running around to all those games and classes but also the impetus behind them that will bring on stress. Trying to meet goals, whether realistic or not, brings on stress.

Frustration at temporary setbacks or obstacles brings on stress. Failure to attain goals brings on stress.

We're not talking about Garrison Keillor's Lake Wobegon here; where every child is above average. Knowing firsthand the damage that can be wrought by unrealistic goals and expectations, I would recommend strongly that parents try to develop their child's sense of acceptance, both by them and himself.

If a father is interested in sports, that's the direction he is likely to push his child. He is likely to do this even in the face of a lack of interest or lack of talent on the part of the child. Remember, sports should be for most recreation, not life.

As sports are games that are, for many, innately enjoyable, the child may take delight in the game itself. The child might be, rather, enjoying the company and attention of the parent. Guiding the child only in the parents' realm of interests may be a case of selling the child too cheaply.

There is music. There is art. There is history. There is a world out there. There is a universe to explore. Take the child to various museums, to plays, to zoos, to parks, to farms. Travel. If means and opportunity are limited, travel the city or take day trips. If possible, introduce them to the variety that is their country.

The stimulus of a child coming into contact with different cultures does wonders. Let the child explore. Let the child find what is available to them. Let the child discover what is in himself. They may find either a vocation or an avocation, or both. They may avoid spending their life in the drudgery of a pursuit not of their own choosing or chosen from an unnecessarily limited menu of options. That leads to settling, to frustration, to less happiness and more stress.

Stress is everywhere. Stress is powerful. Stress can be more harmful than most will imagine. Don't invite it into your life unnecessarily. Don't impose it on your children. Don't program your children's lives to the exclusion of their world of possibilities.

Well, I see it's time to step down from the pulpit and get on with the science.

The Plastic Brain

Yes, the brain is plastic. Your brain is plastic. I didn't insult you by saying your brain is made of plastic. My brain is plastic. Everyone's brain is plastic. To be plastic means only that it is pliant, capable of being molded, modeled, modified.

The brain is being modified almost constantly. Think about it. You saw something or experienced something yesterday. Today you remember it but that memory wasn't in your brain the day before yesterday. Something in your brain changed. That is plasticity.

That isn't the only way your brain is modified but it is a common way. One would think that it is so obvious that it was considered a given since the study of the brain began. Not so.

Another reason the brain's plasticity comes into play is in addiction. The brain adapts to the foreign substance. By adapting to a drug's presence it then experiences problems at its absence. While a drug may give one a pleasant feeling initially, the process of adapting means that the pleasant feeling diminishes. One then requires an ever greater quantity of that substance to maintain the effect for which the use of the drug was begun. It should be noted that there are substances that addict without requiring such increases in dosage. That is just another manifestation of the brain's complexity.

Scientists really didn't accept plasticity of the brain until the early 1980s. Even then neurogenesis was denied by most. Neurogenesis is the creation of new brain cells, synapses and more. It is the fundamental part of plasticity.

I was browsing the NIMH web site in 2003 and came across a page that listed various discoveries and such during that agency's existence. It noted that neurogenesis was first shown in 1983, in large song birds. It was fifteen years later before it was considered likely, by the NIMH, to take place in human beings. Actually, the physical evidence was there for many years but certain quarters failed to recognize it - your tax dollars at work.

Neurogenesis is involved in far more than memory. Stress shuts down the process of neurogenesis. Why? The more basic, primitive aspect of stress is to prepare us for fight or flight. It is a response dedicated to the survival of the organism, you or me. The allostatic system musters and marshals all its resources for survival. Some processes and functions it deems temporarily unessential. You don't need to waste resources digesting food or stimulating your reproductive system while fighting or fleeing. Neither does the allostatic system consider it necessary to devote resources to growing new brain cells at such a time.

I mentioned the need for preparation to fight or flee as being primitive. The danger represented by a sabertooth tiger isn't the only cause for stress. Modern man is stressed by many events and situations a bit more subtle. These are largely social stresses. Going into overdrive as a response to every stressing factor is neither appropriate nor healthy.

The brain and body have other resources. One way we have of responding subtly is by means of heart period variability or respiratory sinus arrhythmia. It may sound odd to the uninitiated but in a healthy heart and system there is a variable length of time between heartbeats. This is controlled by the vagal brake. The variation gives us a vagal tone. As the brake eases off the heart is freed to respond to stress. As the brake releases the vagal tone decreases. If it works improperly, you will have stress-related problems. Primary care physicians should check the vagal tone of all of their patients.

Stress temporarily reduces the overall production of cells involved in memory and thereby its capacity. However, the brain still learns, particularly activities associated with danger. The capacity to learn and develop the memories associated with fear is still there.

Although the brain is limited by stress, the mechanism still has the ability to protect its basic existence. This suggests that, if it is concentrating so heavily on fear while other learning and memory-making is temporarily limited, we may be seeing a description of paranoia.

The memory of fear is generated in the amygdala. The hippocampus provides the necessary context. For a fear to be useful it must be associated with information such as time and place. Where did you encounter that sabertooth tiger? A memory from the amygdala that fails to involve the hippocampus will be a generalized fear. This gives us some phobias and paranoia.

Why would the hippocampus fail to provide the needed context? There could be damage to it. There could be damage to the amygdala. There could be a faulty connection between the two. It could be the expression or repression of one or more genes that is incorrect. The problem could be hereditary, congenital or brought on by stress.

We see that parts of the brain may be shut down, temporarily or permanently, correctly or incorrectly. The opposite side of that coin is that the brain may try to recruit other resources. If so, the auditory system might be brought in. This could explain the hearing of voices. Brain scans have shown that the auditory system of a person with schizophrenia who is hearing voices that others do not appears to function exactly as though he were perceiving actual sounds.

Whether or not, and to what extent, the auditory system becomes involved could be dependant on the general structure of the normal brain. It could be that some brains are already wired in such a way as to make this recruitment likely. It could be that damage caused by chronic stress or the brain's attempt to deal with it increases the chances of auditory system involvement. Perhaps the "Pavlov's Response," where a sound is clearly associated with an important survival situation, in this case fear rather than food, is indicative of the dedication of reduced resources to the essentials of continued existence.

Glutamate is a neurotransmitter that is intimately involved in different types of learning and memory. While cortisol will reduce the production of memory cells it increases production of the glutamate receptor n-methyl-D-aspartate (NMDA). An increase in NMDA receptors means the brain can learn faster.

Now let's jump to what may seem far afield, sex hormones. Let's consider estrogen. It isn't just for breakfast anymore. It protects against free radicals. It protects memory. Significantly, it induces formation of NMDA receptors in the hippocampus.

Don't jump to the conclusion that taking estrogen is a miracle that will enable you to memorize the complete works of William Shakespeare overnight. The brain is far too complicated to yield to such simplistic conclusions. We simply don't know enough to make such a leap. We need far more information than what we have.

Increasing glutamate is not going to provide us with a miracle either. Too much glutamate kills neurons. That isn't something you want to do too frequently.

Progesterone inhibits the synapses. So, do we flood our systems with estrogen and eliminate progesterone? No. Progesterone has its proper roles also. Both have important roles to play in various situations. We just don't have anywhere near enough information at this point to barge ahead. Miracles don't come easily, outside of al-Pharma's public relations factories.

This is merely my way of emphasizing, once again, that if we proceed on the skimpy knowledge of the present, we are in over our heads, so to speak. We can't find complete and final answers based on our present state of ignorance. Discovering some of the effects of one chemical compound cannot be the foundation of miracle cures, except financial cures for the pharmaceutical industry.

Except for the amount of profits generated, I fail to see the difference in the hype generated over the latest fad diet supplement by get-rich-quick charlatans sending you to the health food store and the marketing of the latest miracle cure for Turbiasis by the get-even-richer-even-quicker pharmaceutical giants sending you to your family practitioner.

Fourteen years of research cannot be condensed into the bounds of this book. The rapid pace of new information coming from the labs of neurophysiologists and neurobiologists doesn't allow for a book to be totally up-to-date and inclusive. I have tried here to give the general reader an impression of what we know and how it fits. Further elaboration would more likely confuse than enlighten.

You may find my periodic refrain on the complexities of the brain and how little we truly understand a bit tiresome. It cannot, however, begin to match my own weariness with the incessant prattling about the simpleminded concept of 'chemical imbalance' that I have endured for nearly half a century. The absurdity of the concept has not prevented it from becoming as deeply and permanently etched in the common perception as the Golden Arches of Ronald McDonald.

Not only does it affect me as fingernails on a chalkboard but, of far greater moment, it has wasted decades of time, misdirected billions of dollars and the untold brainpower of thousands of researchers. This waste has cost countless lives and indescribable misery for millions.

Then again, perhaps I'm just overreacting. After all, I am mentally ill.

Personality Disorders

There are a lot of personality disorders out there that can't be blamed on Turbiasis. You'll start meeting them soon after you pull out of your driveway. You might not even have to go that far. Do you remember looking in the mirror this morning?

Some personality disorders may be annoying, to the individual or those around him. Some may be much more difficult to deal with.

Many of those accompanying Turbiasis are very disruptive. They may alienate others. They may destroy relationships. They may make it impossible to get or hold a job.

Some people speak of personality disorders of Agmina as though they are an innate manifestation of the illness. They speak in such terms as to lead you to believe that they consider them hardwired into the brain or reflecting a problem with serotonin levels. This is another indication that these people are to be avoided and ignored.

Personality develops basically from two sources. One is something you see in all children by the age of two, if not sooner. Some children, too few, are quiet. Others are rowdy. Some are curious. Some are indifferent. This is not the area I have in mind.

The other source might be described as a reaction. Our personality develops as we decide the appropriate ways to react to various stimuli and situations. If someone cuts you off on the highway, do you get angry? Do you give them the international signal of displeasure? Or, do you write it off as a part of daily life?

Everyone reacts, one way or another. How we react is determined in large part by our social environment and how we see ourselves. Lots of love and reassurance during our development will have an impact or how we react. From that flows the other part: how we see ourselves. A dislike for oneself can easily be translated into seeing yourself as disliked by others. Did someone do something you don't like because they don't like you? If you see it that way, it will definitely tend to color your perception of the world and play a role in how you react.

Experiencing abuse, physical, sexual, verbal, emotional or any other kind, during the formative years is unlikely to result in a sunny outlook. The stress from such abuse could trigger Turbiasis. With or without Turbiasis, the abuse requires a reaction. It is understandable if a child makes a poor choice at this point.

Most commonly, Agmina will experience some depression, self-doubt or other negative emotions years before they reach the point of exhibiting a diagnosable case of Turbiasis. The outline of one's personality may be formed before it is known that they have the disease.

It becomes a personality disorder when it interferes with your life. Children are given much more leeway than adults. Some aspects of a child's personality defect may be accepted as cute for awhile. It may be seen as obnoxious but then children are expected to get on our nerves sometimes. Several years ago a psychiatrist stated that all teenagers are sociopaths. He said that adults would be arrested or committed if they behaved as many teenagers do.

Turbiasis, even before you are aware of its presence, causes the development of personality disorders. You have feelings of being different. Children don't want to be different. They want acceptance and see that being different is a barrier to that acceptance. They are not likely to come to an adult to discuss these vague feelings. They will try to deal with them on their own.

The likelihood of finding the best way to deal with these problems on their own is small or nonexistent. As each occasion brings with it another misguided or mistaken approach, the personality is further formed. One may very well have an almost completely formed personality by the time the Turbiasis is recognized.

Another problem for Agmina in developing an appropriate personality is the inheritability factor. If you inherited either the Turbiasis or the susceptibility to it, you probably are influenced by a parent who has their own personality disorder. Such a person is more apt to be an aid in developing one's own disorder than being of help in the development of a healthy personality.

As with Turbiasis itself, there is no pill to correct a personality disorder. The therapist will have to break down and actually talk to the patient. It is difficult to imagine any serious personality disorder that one can cure oneself from. If you are seeing a psychiatrist that spends more time with a prescription pad than discussing your problems, run. He is doing lots of harm and he is doing nothing to help you.

The nature of the beast is that being helpful in the cure of a personality disorder is at least as difficult, if not impossible, for family members or others close to the person. This is a matter best left to others. It is also better left to those with proper training and experience. Curing or overcoming a personality disorder may be more problematical than success with the Turbiasis.

Turbiasis and personality disorders may be joined at the hip but success with Turbiasis does not automatically extend to the other. Even a cure of the disease will leave the personality disorder to be dealt with. It will make it easier but not a foregone conclusion. These are separate issues, each requiring due regard and attention.

I have given this subject far less space than it deserves.

Chapter 12

Do Unto Me

Half of the harm that is done in this world is due to people who want to feel important. They don't mean to do harm but the harm does not interest them.
T.S. Eliot

And as ye would that men should do to you, do ye also to them likewise.
Luke 6:31

How many people have an overwhelming desire to be kidnaped, physically and emotionally abused, deprived of their civil, legal and human rights, subjected to toxic nostrums and imprisoned for an indeterminate period to be arbitrarily decided at some future time, if ever? Come on now. Let me see those hands.

I have tried to come up with another medical problem that can result in imprisonment for up to life. No luck. I have tried to think of another medical problem that can result in legalized assault. No luck. I have tried to find another medical problem that allows physicians to gratuitously do damage to one's body or brain. Again, no luck. People who have reached the age of consent have the right to refuse treatment, except for those with Turbiasis.

We are subject to the whims of courts that have no familiarity with our problem. The courts may call upon someone who, in their ignorance, they consider knowledgeable. Putative experts who consider chemical imbalance a credible theory influence the courts. All of this ignorance becomes the basis for the denial of civil rights and imprisonment.

All of the above used to happen to Agmina back in the unenlightened days of yore. All of the above is happening to Agmina this very day. All of the above is done in the guise of our best interest. I would be willing to wager that most people with a somatic illness are thankful that their malady doesn't engender such concern for their best interest. And yet, many professionals in this field express dismay at the lack of appreciation for their efforts by Agmina.

Take notice of a line graph, one recording events of some volatility. Almost any related to the stock market will serve the purpose. What catches our attention are the extremes, the sharp peaks and valleys, the steep climbs and precipitous falls. Buckets of printers ink, both real and virtual, will note the obvious.

Ofttimes, the graph will try to tell us of other factors involved. There may be a long-term trend of more significance, though less eye-catching. There may be an underlying stability in less glamorous sectors of the economy. But even an awareness of these other facets fails to eliminate the initial perceptions, the emotional reactions to those extremes.

Some of my observations on how Agmina are treated and served will engender less than positive responses from providers. While recognizing that much of this treatment and many of those who serve us are not to be identified with these extremes, we must acknowledge that they do exist and that they strongly color the perceptions and resulting attitudes on both sides.

To what extent they do or do not represent the dominant character of the relationship I do not know. Although personal experience, of a necessarily anecdotal nature, makes me think it more than simply an occasional exception, I do not presume to paint all providers with the same broad strokes, as I would hope they would not see Agmina as some homogeneous mass.

If some find these incidents, situations and attitudes not particularly gratifying, please understand that is not the intent. If they cause one to believe that this represents a general attack on those responsible for serving the Agmina, neither is that the intent. Compared to other illnesses, Turbiasis is less understood and more laden with misconceptions while being consigned to the bottom of society's list of priorities.

Many of the incidents I see strike me the way the extremes of the graphs do. They immediately catch my eye. They will do the same to you. There may be things happening that are not as eye-catching that deserve more notice than they attract but those extremes, however embarrassing, do exist and must be acknowledged.

The needs are so great, while the resources are wholly inadequate. How great? Those we classify as having Turbiasis represent in excess of twenty percent of the population. One in every six attempts suicide. This includes just the big three: depression, manic-depression and schizophrenia. Yet as common as it is, we still find lists of major illnesses that omit it.

In testimony before Congress following World War II, the Director of Selective Service, General Louis Hershey, asserted that it represented the greatest loss of resources during that war. Former Surgeon General Thomas Parran described it as the most devastating of all illnesses.

If indeed it is one of the most common major maladies, the most devastating illness and imposes the greatest loss of resources to our society, surely we have assigned it a high priority. Surely we shower researchers with funding. Surely we recruit the best and the brightest to deal with this scourge. Surely we treat the victims with empathy and respect.

The reality is so glaringly to the contrary that even the most optimistic and naive entertain no hope or expectations of ever seeing a level of societal concern appropriate to the needs.

As unflattering a picture as some of the following will be to the providers of services, if the reality of the magnitude of the problems and the embarrassment they should represent could be admitted and appreciated, there is reason for some hope that providers will have the resources they need to do more than maintain the present shameful level of neglect.

This book will not, by itself, have sufficient power to bring significant change. Providers must stop accepting the fact that they have inadequate funds, facilities, staff and leadership. They must refuse to accept the unacceptable.

Being surrounded by the misery that is Turbiasis takes its toll. Most psychiatric social workers begin their career full of sympathy, if not empathy, full of concern for the afflicted. These people, full of hope, fully expect to make a positive contribution, to improve the lives of people who are in desperate need.

They have paid attention in class. They have mastered the latest theories and techniques. They understand what they have been told will remake a broken life. They know they will be rich only in terms that their bankers will not appreciate. They have an idealism that is nothing but a stale joke to the hustlers in their graduating class who expect to turn their diplomas into gold ingots. Fade out.

Look up these dedicated Good Samaritans five years after they doff their caps and gowns. Are some no longer in the field? What? A majority? How can that be?

Well, how about those that are still there? They must have been the truly committed ones. They must take great pride in almost constant success. They must awaken before the alarm begins to blare, racing with anticipation to get out the door and to the office.

What? That doesn't ring true for those of you who are still in the trenches? You mean the idealism is just an embarrassing memory? Frustration with the illness, frustration with the clients, frustration with the system, frustration after frustration has become the constant, every day that you trudge back to work.

What happened? It really isn't a secret. It really isn't surprising. It is burnout. The lot of those laboring in this field is to daily deal with a world of misery and failure. Hopes are not fulfilled, the idealism of the undergraduate wanes and withers.

It's difficult for those disposed to choose this field for a career not to care about their clients as individuals. Caring becomes a problem. This person you are trying to help doesn't magically respond to treatment. This person may become worse. This person may not believe he is ill. This person may, in a fit of paranoia, even see you as his tormentor.

The resources are not available. A desperately needed bed at a group home or institute will require getting on a waiting list. Into jail or out on the street, this person you care about is losing the battle. You feel guilty. You feel inadequate. You no longer feel you are making any difference. You feel the stress. You wonder why you can't help this person whose well-being defines your success, indeed, the career choice you made all those years ago.

It isn't just one of those for whom you are responsible. It is several, or most, or all. You've invested too much in this career. You've lost your own belief in yourself, your ability to transition to another line of work. You're stuck. These people never appreciated your efforts or wouldn't do their part. Why should you care? No one else seems to. Why should you take that frustration home with you every night? You're burned out. What are your options?

Your options may be to get out, stay and just go through the motions or get away from the personal contact by playing the corporate game, getting promoted out of casework. One option you don't have is to continue to care. It may be a conscious decision. It may not. It doesn't matter. You have to stop caring, for your own self-protection. You just can't take the heartbreak anymore. You can't take the frustration, the failure or the stress any longer.

Giving up requires distancing yourself from these people. If you cannot or will not distance yourself physically, you must do so emotionally. It's not just a passive development. It isn't they who are changing. It's you. They are staying in the same place. You are the one actively putting a distance between them and your feelings for them.

This distancing is not simple and it is not without consequences. It requires you to strip yourself of the emotional attachments you once had. It doesn't allow you to think of them as individuals, as personalities any longer.

At best they become a bit less than fellow human beings. They become objects. It becomes a case of us and them. They become your adversaries, your opponents, your enemies. They become an intrusion on your life. Don't let them create problems for you. Just shut them up.

Do some providers, those being paid to help and care for the Agmina, really abuse their charges? Do politicians have egos? It happens.

Some studies have had more than one-third of the respondents admit to physical abuse. How many did the deed but failed to admit to it? We really don't know how pervasive such abuse is. We just know that it is not rare.

Who Cares?

Back in the mid-nineties, within a space of five months, in one state institution, three patients were raped. Each victim was a male patient in his early twenties. One victim was raped by three other patients. The incident lasted approximately one hour. It happened on a Gurney next to a nursing station.

How did the staff and administration respond to this heinous crime? The victim was put into an isolation cell, without food, without water, without access to toilet facilities until he was prepared to sign a statement asserting that he was a willing participant.

The father of one, a retired official with the Federal Bureau of Investigation, was incensed. He protested to the administrator of the institute. He protested to the commissioner of the state department of mental health. He protested to the chief of police, the mayor, anyone. He was always met with the statement that his son was coerced into signing. No corrective action. No apologies. No show of concern. No penalties. No redress. No justice.

The young man was in the institute because he was in a traumatized state. The rape represented a further trauma. He was still further traumatized by the isolation cell and the pressure to admit to a lie which branded him as a homosexual. He then shared the frustration of his father's futile efforts at redress. Would you have difficulty seeing him being driven to the brink of suicide?

All of this resulted from the action and inaction of providers, from the people paid and sworn to help him. What he encountered was a group of providers who were more concerned with not upsetting their lives - at any cost to their ward. These were human beings one would expect to feel some empathy for a victim under their care and protection. Such expectations would have been sadly unrealized.

I mentioned three incidents. The salient differences in the other two cases were that there was only one assailant and the families of those victims were poor and limited their protests to the institute's administration and the police. They obviously fared no better.

Mentioning three incidents does not exhaust the scores of such serious complaints I have been called on to help with. We would prefer to think that these incidents are rare. They aren't. They are far more common than is reported. We would like to think that these incidents are relics of the past. They aren't. Similar atrocities are taking place while you read this page.

These responses could not have occurred had the providers seen these victims as people, had they seen them as fellow citizens. They would not have exhibited such callous disregard for the victims had they been cancer patients in a general hospital.

My perspective may be colored by my experience but I find it difficult to believe that the treatment these young men received was unrelated to their condition.

As executive director of a nonprofit advocacy organization, a large part of our funding came from federal grants. It was far from adequate but we were in no position to decline the funds with any expectation of the organization surviving. The average income of the membership was about half of the amount that the federal government considered the poverty level. The ten dollar annual dues had to be waived for most of the membership.

We had to endure the insult of not being considered capable of handling the funds ourselves. This attitude persisted despite the fact that both the average educational attainments and management experience of the organization's office staff was considerably greater than that of the state department handling the funds. The money was funneled through the state department of mental health.

We were assured that the arrangement was merely an administrative convenience. They were unable to point to other organizations, unrelated to Turbiasis, that labored under such administrative arrangements. We were assured that the funds were ours to use within the framework of the federal guidelines and without interference by the state. And Santa Claus lays Easter eggs.

There were problems however. We took our organization's *raison d'etre* seriously. We actually advocated on behalf of our membership.

As the department, and its commissioner, were the same ones involved in denying redress to the above-mentioned victims of rape in one of its own institutes, it should not be surprising that our advocacy did not sit well with that department.

The rapes and the department's handling of them were not the problem. The problem was that we chose not to ignore their malfeasance, misfeasance and nonfeasance.

Our ungrateful attitude on this and many other matters did not go unnoticed. We were constantly the target of intimidation and insult. The department made every attempt to micro-manage our independent, membership organization of Agmina. The department would order officials of the organization to come to the department.

Factotums of the department would tell the board when to meet. They would tell the board where to meet. They demanded meetings include their staff. Their staff members would interrupt the organization's representatives to change the topic if it was one that offended them. One could easily get the impression that these state officials were more comfortable with a plantation mentality than one would expect well over a century after the Emancipation Proclamation.

In Prison

A basic problem of our prison systems is that we, the public, don't know what we want them to do. Should they protect us by keeping bad people off the streets? Should they punish these bad people? Should they wreak revenge for us good people? Should they rehabilitate their charges? We don't speak with one voice. We send confusing messages to those in charge of the systems. We change the message or the emphasis. We have the worst of all possible situations for trying to develop a rational approach.

I have some opinions on what a rational approach should be but this is not the place to burden you with them. That said, there are a couple of general observations that need to be aired. These lead to a little story about one inmate with Turbiasis.

Over ninety percent of those in prison will get out. The major outcomes of our present ways of handling this population are to make reentry into society unlikely of success and to provide an education in the development of criminal skills. These are not the intended consequences but, nevertheless, they are also the unarguable consequences.

The most powerful tools available for enhancing the chances of successful reentry are the visitation programs. Prison officials commonly screw these up. Even the best systems I am aware of fail to maximize their potential. Keeping in touch with the outside world, through substantive contact and interaction with family and friends makes the outside seem more real and more achievable.

The way visitation programs are usually set up is as a method of control for the benefit of the staff. The visitation program becomes a system of reward and punishment rather than a positive tool to reduce recidivism and provide the inmates and the community a chance at success. Yes, I've read the policy statements. They say many of the right words. In the real world they are nothing more than window dressing.

Visiting with family and friends can bring about a considerable reduction in the level of stress. Prison is, by its very nature, stressful. There is no way to eliminate it but visitation and other efforts can reduce it. Anything, within the bounds of security, that can be done to reduce stress will be of enormous importance to Agmina.

How it Really Works

A bit of orientation would probably be helpful to those unfamiliar with penal and legal systems. Most prisoners are provided periodic parole hearings. Depending on a host of variables, these may occur annually or somewhat less frequently. Parole should not be expected at most of these hearings. Often, the hearing is strictly *pro forma,* going through the motions for appearance sake and to satisfy the legal requirements. Sometimes the hearing is part of building a record for later hearings, when parole is more probable.

I received a phone call late one afternoon. An inmate in a facility about 150 miles away was thought by others to be potentially suicidal. He had been scheduled for a parole hearing. Why was he suicidal?

The rules require a drug test prior to a hearing. A couple of days prior to the hearing the inmate is awakened in the wee hours, given a cup and expected to produce a sample while two guards watch. The rule states that, if no sample is given within a certain time frame, it is put down as a failed drug test. The results of a failed drug test are a cancellation of the hearing, a serious black mark on one's permanent record, a stretch in 'the hole,' solitary confinement, and loss of their visitation privileges.

Why didn't he produce a sample? He suffers from Turbiasis. He is HIV positive. He is severely underweight. So? First, let's address the weight. In such a situation there are less body fluids. Dehydration is a consideration.

The regulation of body fluids is just one of the several functions of the cholinergic system. Substances that are intended to reduce the fluid levels are termed anti-cholinergic. Although some medications may be intended for other purposes, they may have an anti-cholinergic side effect. Would you believe that most, if not all, medications for depression and HIV have that side effect? It's true. As noted earlier, stress, through the allostatic system, can have an effect on the cholinergic system. He was definitely experiencing stress.

Solitary confinement would have to wait a few days. Even though the prison staff was putting two inmates into each 'solitary' cell, there was a waiting list.

I was asked to intervene during this interval. A call was made to the deputy warden, a nice man. He listened to my reasons and set aside the solitary confinement. The problem was that the hearing was rescheduled for a couple of weeks later. This required another drug test.

Another test. Another failure. Another sentence to solitary. Another call. A different outcome. The warden took the case away from her deputy, even though such matters were designated as a part of the deputy's portfolio.

When objection was made to sending him to solitary, on the basis of the anti-cholinergic effects of his medications, the warden asked the staff physician for his opinion. Her report to the commissioner included the physician's opinion that the medications did interfere with urination but still her recommendation was that the inmate be put in solitary and otherwise punished anyway. The commissioner agreed. Don't ask me why. My guess is a couple of petty people showing off their power.

One would think that the specter of all the paperwork required for a suicide would have given these bureaucrats pause. It may be giving them too much credit to think that crossed their minds. But why would they take a chance with someone's life? Weren't there other options? Yes. The drug test could have been accomplished with blood or hair analysis. They could have asked the guards of his unit. The guards, as well as other inmates, know who are on drugs and who aren't.

Being in solitary didn't but could have brought on a suicide attempt. The young man was fragile, on the edge. It was said by one inmate it was possible he may have gathered strength from the knowledge that someone cared when the initial intervention spared him.

Our thoughts during this period quite naturally were focused on preventing suicide but, absent suicide, we need to deal with the punishment that followed: denial of visitation for a year. Beyond the convenience of the staff in having one more tool for control, or the pleasure that some individuals obviously derive in causing suffering to others, particularly those who are helpless, visitation is a potentially powerful tool for the benefit of both society and the inmate themselves.

Inmates, in general, but those with Turbiasis, particularly, are paying a heavy price. Society also is paying a heavy price for such shortsighted policies and the indulgence of a number of prison officials and staff in their perversions.

A large proportion of the mental health services in prisons are directed to dealing with substance abuse. This is true to a lessor extent on the outside. The volatile admixture of a problem such as depression with alcohol or drug abuse complicates the delivery system for services and the situation for the individual patient.

With this new model, we can see that some addictions and some aspects of addiction need to fall within the bounds of Turbiasis. Substance abuse can be a stand-alone malady under this heading. Another matter we must deal with is dual diagnosis. This refers to someone having one of the traditional illnesses and substance abuse, concurrently.

We need to be careful with dual diagnosis. From my observations and experience, the substance abuse more commonly should not be classified as an addiction in the strict sense. It is more likely to be an habituation. The use of alcohol or drugs by a person with depression, for instance, usually is a case of self-medication. The person feels bad and uses the substance to feel better.

The last paragraph in no way is intended to minimize the problem of substance abuse. It is meant to put it in proper perspective when associated with depression or its brethren. Even if it is an habituation, it still represents a problem that will require attention. The depression is the root problem, however, and needs to be seen as the more critical matter.

I usually see treatment primarily directed at the substance abuse with the other as somewhat of an afterthought. In a dual diagnosis case there will be little or no progress made on either front when the substance abuse is the chief point of focus.

Regardless of the reasons for abuse of Agmina, they suffer from it. Whether it results from a provider who is burnt out, from the lack of adequate resources, from someone who delights in the discomfiture of others or from a system that is irrational, the burden is borne by the Agmina.

Chapter 13

Penny Wise and Pound Foolish

For I was an hungred, and ye gave me meat: I was thirsty, and ye gave me drink: I was a stranger, and ye took me in: Naked, and ye clothed me: I was sick, and ye visited me: I was in prison, and ye came unto me.

The righteous ask when they had done these deeds for him and he responded: Verily I say unto you, Inasmuch as ye have done it unto one of the least of these my brethren, ye have done it unto me.

To the others, he said: Depart from me, ye cursed, into everlasting fire,
Matthew 25:35-41

Never attribute to malice that which can be adequately explained by stupidity.
Anonymous

I speak for the Least of These. Let's look for a bit at those who are supposed to represent the interests of the Agmina. I'm going to focus on just a fraction of the problem, as the total numbers for the entire society are too large to fully comprehend or appreciate. The numbers, unless otherwise noted, come from a presentation made in the early nineteen-nineties to a state's joint legislative health committee.

As with most political subdivisions of our nation, they were wringing their hands over a number of budget problems. When you have a budget problem, you don't start including those items which would be nice to have. You don't, or shouldn't, even begin with needs. You set priorities. You begin with that which is vital.

Health is vital. The most tragic realm of health is Turbiasis. It is tragic because of the illness itself. It is tragic because of our society's failure to do that which is doable. It is tragic because of its ramifications for the whole of society.

One family in four is affected by Turbiasis. Repeated studies have shown it to be growing faster than the general population.

How horrible is Turbiasis to contemplate? A survey taken in the 1960s ranked it second only to leprosy among the most feared of illnesses. Since then, leprosy has fallen off our screens.

I have known three individuals who were plagued with both Turbiasis and blindness. There was another friend who has been in a wheelchair with scoliosis for nearly forty years. All stated unequivocally that Turbiasis was their most difficult burden to bear.

Turbiasis is a disease that is second to none in numbers, in costs, in duration, in disruption of lives. What has been the response at the state level, on the national level?

Compared to the 1960s, the state reduced the number of beds at the institutes by more than 85 percent. This one savings alone amounted to more than half a billion dollars a year by the mid-nineties, a multiple of the present state budget for all services to the Agmina.

Adjust for inflation and you are likely speaking of something in excess of two billion of today's dollars. Factor in population growth for a period of three or four decades. It is obvious that, even in one small state, we are having to deal with staggering numbers.

I said the reduction of beds represented a savings of more than half a billion dollars *per annum* in a relatively small state. I was wrong. I simply don't know how to calculate all of the collateral costs, even the ones which might be quantified in dollars. The calculation of the costs in lives, the costs in pain, in misery and anguish, the costs in crime, the cost in human resources for this one state alone is well beyond the capacity of all that state's computing power.

Where Are Our Leaders?

If more than 1,000,000 citizens of that state suffered the temporary losses associated with fire, drought, flood, earthquake or pestilence, the governor would immediately declare a state of emergency.

For the Least of These the losses tend to be permanent and growing. Where is the governor? Where is his call for those in Washington to send the desperately needed assistance? Where is the legislature? Do they not realize the disaster in their own little bailiwicks?

Are these 1,000,000-plus souls unimportant? Is their grief, their pain, their suffering of so little note or concern of these officials? Obviously, but why? Is it acceptable to ignore the devastation of their lives because they committed the crime of being born with or developing Turbiasis?

You have undoubtedly heard many ideas for reducing crime. Permit me to suggest a guaranteed way.

The FBI tells us that of the general population seven percent will commit a crime of violence qualifying as a felony. Among Agmina it is two percent. Of that two percent, most is self-directed as suicide or self-mutilation. Over in England the respective figures were seven percent and three percent.

Remember back in Chapter 7 where we learned of the effects of withdrawal from medication? Remember akathisia?

A study was done by the National Institute for Mental Health of the levels of crime committed by those Agmina who were released from institutes without follow-up care. This category was twice as likely to commit murder, five times as likely to commit aggravated assault, seven times as likely to commit rape and eight times as likely to commit robbery as the general population. Compare this to the overall population of Agmina and to the general population.

Is this violent group of Agmina, released from institutes without follow up care a significant part of the population? Not as a percentage of the whole but it is a major factor in specific segments. Every estimate of the percentage of the homeless with Turbiasis ranges from one-third to one-half.

The largest institute for the Agmina was once New York's Pilgrim Institute with a population of around 3,000. Presently, the institute housing the greatest number of Agmina is the Los Angeles County Jail. It averages at least 3,500.

If the institutes designed for this population, staffed with people supposedly trained in this specialty were so unsuccessful, what should we expect from life on the street or from personnel trained as jailers? The trend and the results are not peculiar to any one city, state or region. There is no place immune to the entirely predictable results of kicking people out of the institutes without care.

State and national legislators, administrators and executives somehow seem convinced that the half billion dollars saved in that one small state has no untoward effects. They think it has no effect beyond making more funds available for less critical budget items or giving a tax cut or saving their own political rears by obviating the need for spending tax dollars on people they consider less than human.

Chapter 14

A Bitter Pill

Any party which takes credit for the rain must not be surprised if its opponents blame it for the drought.
Dwight Morrow

A business that makes nothing but money is a poor business.
Henry Ford

Examine what is said, not him who speaks.
Arabian Proverb

Fair and balanced were generally considered positive words until recently, when they became besmirched by being reduced to the level of an ironic advertising and marketing phrase.

However positive their connotations, they are frequently mutually exclusive. The truth may not please everyone but it is, by and large, deemed fair, though many don't want it spoken.

Balanced, as used in a political context, is commonly unfair. Politics is defined as the relationship between two or more individuals or groups. In this sense the subject of this chapter is political. It covers the actions of the drug lords and the medical establishment as they relate to the rest of us, as individuals and as groups.

In 2003, Paul Krugman, economist, professor, author and columnist for the *New York Times* gave a talk. He discussed the term balanced. He asked us to suppose that the President made a statement that the world was flat. He suggested that a 'balanced' headline might read, "Shape of the Earth in Question."

For educated people in the 21st Century, indeed, most everyone, that would be seen as nonsense. But, balance would require putting such a statement on the same level as fact. Such a headline would not be fair to the truth, to reduce it to that level, just for the sake of balance.

Putting truth and facts on a par with falsehoods and ignorance is unfair. It would be an ill-advised quest, to attempt balancing the unbalanced. Powerful interests commonly demand that any criticism of their position be balanced. al-Pharma spends billions of dollars fostering their mono-themed messages, promoting themselves and their products without balance, but cry foul if anyone displays the temerity to offer an opposing view. If their cries of complaint about a lack of balance are insufficient, they then attack the messenger.

Peter Breggin attacked the American Psychiatric Association and was accused of being a mouthpiece for Scientology. It was untrue but truth is seldom an obstacle for determined people when their gravy train is threatened. As for me, I consider Scientology a scam more than a cult. I had an employee in Los Angeles back in the 1960s who was a member and whose father was an official of the group. As he related its precepts, it seemed ludicrous even then.

The one point of commonality, opposition to psychiatry, is all that we share, and that for disparate reasons. I see psychiatry, as it relates to Turbiasis, intellectually fraudulent and very harmful to the interests of Agmina. Scientology sees psychiatry as competition. Psychiatrists may engage in all of the marriage counseling they wish. I won't care. Scientology can finance all of the *Battlefield Earth*-type movies they wish. I don't care, but people with Turbiasis should stay as far away as possible from both.

There was a recent dustup between Scientology and psychiatry. Actor Tom Cruise made an ill-advised comment about Brooke Shield's use of an antidepressant and her flackery on behalf of the drug industry. Neither did a service to the public. Scientology, relying on what it calls Dianetics, claims to "clear" the brain. It therefore sees psychiatry as competition. They provide their adherents with ammunition against psychiatry. Much of their criticism is accurate. That doesn't make them the final authority on the mind, however. That doesn't prove their approach to be valid.

I have every sympathy for Brooke Shield's struggle with postpartum depression. But that ordeal does not qualify her as an expert. It does not justify her writing a book advising all other women experiencing that problem to take a pill.

Antidepressants are chemically similar to cocaine and amphetamines. They all inhibit the reuptake of serotonin. Cocaine and amphetamines are classified as stimulants. Studies report that 10 to 25% of those on Prozac experienced the stimulant effect. If you feel depressed, a stimulant, with a concomitant increase in energy level, is likely to be interpreted as making you feel better. The person taking the drug is not usually the best judge of their state. Try taking the car keys from a drunk. He'll probably see himself as fully capable of driving. He may put up a fight. I would hope that you would not accept his self-assessment as gospel. The effects of a drug may color one's judgment. You know that.

An increase in energy may cause one to feel better but it does not mean that the depression is relieved. It ignores the damage being done to the brain. Tom's criticism of Brooke was off-putting to quite a few people. A little knowledge is a dangerous thing. Perhaps it would have been better for him not to broach the subject.

Brooke's role as an expert, advising others to follow her lead, was a disaster of miscasting. A little knowledge is a dangerous thing. Someone said that already, didn't they?

The attack on Peter Breggin is reminiscent of General Motors and Ralph Nader in the 1960s. The automotive giant felt threatened by Nader's book about the Corvair, *Unsafe at Any Speed*. They hired private investigators. The only dirt they could come up with were citations for reckless or drunken driving. There was just one minor problem. It was completely fabricated.

Crusader Ralph didn't own a car and never had. He never had a drivers license. A friend was killed in an accident when he was young, so he opted never to drive. General Motors had egg on its face and had to issue an apology. Their willingness to ignore the truth and engage in an *ad hominem* attack on the messenger, rather than challenge the message with fact, was not only an embarrassment for them but helped build Nader's platform.

Given the realities of the publishing business, it is unlikely that this book will attain sufficient notice to prompt any response from the pharmaceutical or medical industries. If it were to receive even a fraction of the attention a book such as Nader's drew, the long knives would be unsheathed.

Although there might be an attempt to discredit the message, the facts on which it is based are well-documented. Any fight on that front would provide a free platform for the particulars they want to suppress and give the public a chance to see what has been drowned out by their billions of dollars of marketing.

More likely, there would be a personal attack, directing attention away from the message. I may be characterized as someone on the fringe, as one of those who deny there is such a thing as Turbiasis. Absolutely untrue. I know it from five decades of firsthand experience and a bit more at secondhand through family members, friends and thousands I have met as an advocate and in other capacities.

I may be portrayed as a Luddite, as one who denies all of the advances of modern science. Nothing could be further from the truth. I can easily pull out the copies of my patents. Based on their past behavior there is no expectation they will own up to their culpability. We are not dealing with normal people here; not normal in the sense that they are, socially, ethically, developmentally immature.

Show Me the Money

al-Pharma seemingly owns the alphabet. It owns the FDA, the NIMH, the APA, the AMA and NAMI. Beyond those it owns the government. It is the largest lobbying group in the country by any measure. They have more lobbyists on Capitol Hill than there are legislators, at least 100 more. They own the majority of our Representatives and Senators by far.

Paul Krugman points out that the Medicare pharmacy bill, written by the drug industry's law/lobbying firm in their offices, was shepherded through Congress by Billy Tauzin, a 'representative' from Louisiana.

Little Billy immediately left Congress to head the Pharmaceutical Research and Manufacturers of America, al-Pharma. He warns us that allowing drugs to be imported at cheaper prices would give al-Qaeda the opportunity to import anthrax as fake Viagra. Wow! I never thought of that! Wasn't the anthrax scare that caused the evacuation of Congress from the good ole US of A, Billy?

Krugman further notes that Thomas Scully, former Medicare administrator, threatened to fire the chief actuary if he didn't hide the true cost of the Medicare pharmacy bill. He then received a waiver from ethics rules to permit him to negotiate a lobbying job with the health industry while pushing the drug bill. Man, is this a great country, or what?

As many have noted, this is more than a corrupt person here and another one over there. It is a corrupt system.

From the point of view of research, the pharmaceutical companies are basically stuck in the 1950s. That decade gave us neuroleptics, monoamine oxidase inhibitors and tricyclics. They still offer us this unholy trinity.

According to the FDA, they have not developed any medications that are more effective, but they have made amazing progress in marketing a multitude of clones. Present drug categories provide such massive profits while requiring minimal research costs that they are unlikely to stop cranking out xerox drugs. The only way to stop it is to cease issuing patents for drugs unless they represent something new, efficacious and safe— as the law requires.

Elsewhere in this book I have outlined the limitations and drawbacks of the trinity. They are ineffective and seriously damaging to the people afflicted by Turbiasis, however profitable they might be for others. More than that, the obsession with the profits to be made from these artifacts of ignorance from the middle of the last century divert resources from the proven therapies and research that at least hold the promise of progress.

I have suggested lines of inquiry elsewhere in this book that hold varying degrees of promise. Some fall within the purview of the pharmaceutical companies, academic researchers and the NIMH. They are not, as present research, based on counterfactual premises. They are a direct result of looking at the facts, organizing them, finding a common thread, applying logic and trying to start from the inside and work outward, instead of starting with attacks on the observable symptoms.

I feel as though I have opened a door in a darkened room and entered a room lit with a single candle. Once my eyes adjusted I could clearly see several doors, many with gaps around the edges showing the promise of brightly lit rooms on the other side.

I will entertain no criticism from al-Pharma or those beholden to them. They have no scientific basis for their position. To argue with ignorance and intentional error is simply a waste. At my age I have little enthusiasm for spending any of the remainder of my time engaging those charlatans in pointless debate.

This different perspective doesn't have the billions of dollars of marketing behind it. To expect me, with extremely limited resources and opportunities to balance this effort by also repeating the nonsense the reader has been inundated with for decades is unfair. If my meager efforts can cause these multibillion-dollar conglomerates to fret, they must be more aware than I how flimsy is the house of cards upon which the 'chemical imbalance' model depends.

The foregoing was intended to be the preamble to a fair (truthful) but unbalanced attack on al-Pharma, on grounds not covered elsewhere in the book. Marcia Angell, in her book, *The Truth About the Drug Companies,* made much of this chapter unnecessary. There are, however, a couple of areas that she covers on which I do wish to comment.

al-Pharma spends unbelievable amounts on the promotion of certain of their products. Sometimes it is called advertising. Sometimes it is called marketing. Sometimes it is called education. All of the time it is an unnecessary waste.

Advertising wasn't needed to tell the world about the polio vaccine. Most people have never heard of Taxol. Why? Physicians quickly got the word that an effective drug for some types of cancer was available.

For a polio vaccine, the public needed to know of its existence. The media informed them. Taxol was not a preventive medicine, so only segments of the medical community needed to know. Advertising was unneeded in both cases. It was not needed because the medications were needed.

If you see advertising for a drug, it means that it is an unnecessary medication. It may be less effective than other drugs or classes of drugs. It may be in competition with several other drugs that are distinguishable only by brand name, color, shape, price and/or ad campaign.

If you see advertising for a drug, don't buy it. You will be paying for the advertising and getting screwed. If you see advertising for a drug, it means it cannot stand on its own merits.

Marketing is for the company's benefit, not yours. As Ms. Angell points out, when Eli Lilly's patent for Prozac expired, they created a new medical problem. They called it premenstrual dysphoric disorder. They received approval from the FDA to market it for this new 'disorder.' They changed the color. They changed the name, Sarafem. They changed the price. They increased it from that of Prozac when it was protected by patent. They sold it for more than three times the price of the generic substitutes for the newly patent-bare Prozac.

What benefit does the sucker, er uh, customer get from paying more for the same ingredients from the same manufacturer? Remember that these ingredients provably didn't alleviate or cure depression when sold as Prozac and there is no evidence to prove that they provide any benefit to anyone suffering from PMS. Paying more will make Mr. Lilly happy but is unlikely to improve the product's performance.

Resorting to Education

Education is, or is supposed to be, objective. al-Pharma's promotion of its products is not objective. al-Pharma's promotion of its products is not education, regardless of what they call it.

I also haven't grasped the necessity for the education of practicing physicians to be combined with all-expense paid vacations to Hawaii or Las Vegas or Broadway or Hilton Head. Are these learned gentlemen incapable of absorbing information outside the confines of a resort? Are the costs of all these festivities not paid for out of the pockets of their patients? Are they entitled to this largess at our expense?

Even more than the burden of the extra costs to their patients is the mind set this education generates. The industry has taken over the pharmaceutical education of physicians from medical school to retirement. The result is that medical students are imbued with a pronounced predilection to reach for the prescription pad as their first and, far too frequently, only option. This is the sad truth in many specialties but particularly in the treatment of Turbiasis.

A great deal of money is directed at educating the public. As with all of their purported educational efforts, all of their advertising to the public is at best misleading. Zoloff ads are a fraud. Cartoon figures, little circles with frowns, then smiles, were used to front the message that depression may be the result of chemical imbalance.

A later use of these same little characters, in a remarkably similar looking advertisement with nearly the same copy, was pushing its value in dealing with anxiety. Then it was used again to boast its effectiveness for treating social anxiety disorder.

The word 'may' was carefully chosen, for legal reasons. They know that it isn't true. It is interesting that, while the message begins with that iffy 'may,' it finishes with a line to the effect that you can do something about the malady, disease, disorder, whatever, when you know what is causing it. How do they get from 'may' to 'know' so easily?

The culpability of al-Pharma is complimented by that of the medical industry. Physicians are enjoying the benefits of their having been co-opted. They have allowed the drug companies to set the price at which they can be bought.

While many physicians are traipsing around a world-class golf course or sharing a night on Broadway with their spouse, their patients are tolerating the effects of their disease, dealing with the side effects of their prescriptions and paying exorbitant prices to subsidize those freebies. One estimate puts the value of gifts, honoraria and other forms of bribery and kickbacks at an average per physician of somewhere above $20,000 annually.

There is no evidence that the drug lords have any interest in helping Agmina or any other potential customer. There is overwhelming evidence that they are willing to do anything to suck another buck out of us. Not alone of course, they have played a major role in corrupting our system. No group needs 100 more lobbyists than there are legislators in the Capitol. Just as with their marketing and their products, their strategy is overkill.

The court records, along with mountains of other evidence, shows their willingness to steal from the government, insurance companies, customers, anyone and everyone. The record is filled with their lies. The record shows their complete disregard for playing by the rules. They violate strictures on what they are allowed to claim for their products, both as to what it can be used for and its effectiveness.

al-Pharma hides information from the FDA, the medical community and the public in order to sell products they know to be harmful, even unto death. Are we to play oh so nicely and refrain from calling a thief 'a thief' while they are committing their acts of thievery? Are we supposed to behave civilly towards them while they are poisoning us?

I am assured of receiving criticism for such comments. I didn't make this up. It's all out there in the records. Those who can criticize someone for repeating such important matters in a defense of these miscreants should answer a few questions as to their own reasons.

Chapter 15

Requiem

A man's dying is more the survivors' affair than his own.
Thomas Mann

I didn't attend the funeral, but I sent a nice letter saying I approved of it.
Mark Twain

The medical specialty of bloodletting has declined somewhat of late. The science of phrenology has also fallen on hard times. Exorcism still feeds off of a slowly dwindling number of credulous victims. Easy come. Easy go.

Based on almost as credible a scientific foundation as the above scams, psychiatry seems headed to the same section of the museum.

The next generation of students on their field trips can giggle at the quaintness of the exhibits:

"Yo. Look at this. They actually thought wiggling a big needle around in some dude's skull was scientific."

"Were they stupid enough to really believe that frying someone's brain helped?"

"At least those snake oil salesmen over in the last room sold them something that got 'em drunk. How did they sweet-talk people into taking these little poison pills?"

"It's hard to believe anyone could be so cruel to sick people."

"Okay, class. You're assignment is to explain why they did this. Was it malice, greed or ignorance? Make a case for the one you think it is."

"Teacher? What if we think it was for a combination of those?"

Psychiatry has betrayed the Hippocratic Oath, its own *raison d'etre* and its patients in a desperate attempt to embrace money, prestige and power. This is reflective of a deep-seated insecurity, a collective inferiority complex. I'm just dabbling in a bit of role-reversal here.

Wannabees

Psychiatry was treated as a redheaded stepchild by the rest of the medical community for a very long time. Psychiatrists hungered for acceptance. They have realized that their salvation lay in being able to offer treatment of a somewhat somatic nature. Talk was considered cheap.

In their desperation, psychiatrists were willing to latch on to anything that came down the pike. There were all the various water tortures. There were beatings. There were operations to rid the patients of the organ of the month. There were the lobotomies.

Modern times brought electricity. So, electric shock was their answer. The 'real' physicians were latching on to drugs. "Let's give them a try." Here came acids, laxatives, insulin shock therapy, hallucinogens, whatever. It didn't matter what it did to the patient. It only mattered that it held out the hope that the specialty might be taken seriously by the others in the medical profession.

Did any of these lunatic therapies work? Sure. If you don't understand how they could work, don't feel lonesome. The psychiatrists rarely bothered with explanations or theories, at least rational ones. That didn't hold them back, though. Most of these therapies worked at least ninety percent of the time. Some brought cures. Others only made the patients better. How do we know? They told us so.

Why don't we use these miracle cures now? It appears I forgot to teach you one of the fundamental principles of psychiatric practice. When a new miracle arrives on the scene, all preceding miracles cease to work. I'm not certain as to why this is so but I guess it would be discourteous not to allow the new treatment to bask in an unshared spotlight, to get its share of the pie.

It's possible that there is an element of marketing consideration involved. It is wiser to have something to distract everyone's attention from the stories starting to circulate about the predecessor. A time-honored tradition in the profession, it lives on today in undiminished glory.

Taking away their prescription pads and their electric shock equipment will deprive them of their primary pillars of support. No longer being able to scribble on the prescription pads, they might have to cut back on those free golfing vacations and nights out on Broadway. As kindhearted as al-Pharma may be, I doubt they will continue to dole out quite as much largesse to a group that no longer is poisoning their patients.

The American Psychiatric Association would have to go on welfare were it to anger the drug companies. Over 30 percent of their budget comes from the advertising in their journals. More of their budget comes from the same sources in other forms. Their members enjoy honorariums, vacations, subsidized conferences and numerous other goodies.

Both as individuals and as a group, they have been bought and paid for. They are caught in a golden cage. From inside that cage it appears impossible for them to discern any conflicts of interest. The well-being of their patients may be out there somewhere but has never been high on their list of priorities.

I shouldn't give anyone the impression that the psychiatric profession is totally oblivious to their patients. That would be unfair. When their failure to warn patients of such problems as tardive dyskinesia, as required by law, resulted in a wave of successful lawsuits, rising into the millions of dollars, the APA finally did send a warning letter to their membership.

It would not be very kind of me to leave you with the impression that the APA and the bulk of its members are merely avaricious charlatans.

I have tried to emulate Diogenes in my quest to find an honest psychiatrist. After 14 years of research and firsthand and secondhand experience spreading out over more than half a century, I am almost empty-handed.

Perhaps they are hiding their lights under a bushel. It would be nice if the Southern Baptists, or some other denomination, could send representatives to a few APA conventions and seminars to teach them the words to the song, *This Little Light of Mine*.

Without their prescription pads, most people will see no advantage for the psychiatrists over the psychologists. They will see the higher prices charged by the former. What will the psychiatrists say about their rivals then?

Who's Qualified to Harm Us?

Many psychologists recently have been clamoring for the right to prescribe. Yes, foolish but true. Even though they propose limiting themselves to psychopharmaceuticals and requiring a considerable amount of training in pharmacy, the psychiatrists scoff that psychologists would still be grossly unqualified, dangerous, in fact. Perhaps psychiatrists do have a sense of irony, if not humor.

Now let's look at the other side. Psychiatrists would not dare to question the qualifications of other physicians, even though they have essentially no training in psychiatry, psychology or psychopharmacology. Remember, they are desperate for acceptance by the community of physicians. Even podiatrists have prescribed Prozac. So have a number of veterinarians. One wouldn't want their left big toe to begin behaving irrationally; nor their poodle, for that matter.

While physicians in other specialties are writing eighty percent of the psychiatric prescriptions, stealing their patients, psychiatrists focus their efforts on battling psychologists. One questions their logic when a drug company circulates a twenty-five question, eight and one-half minute test to the non-psychiatric physicians that assures them of being able to correctly diagnose Turbiasis. Can we guess what treatment they offer?

The shrinks would have you believe that all, untrained physicians are magically transformed by this little test into qualified practitioners with pads. Is psychiatry that easy? It's confusing.

Psychiatrists are telling us that someone with a doctorate in psychology and a rigorous course in psychoactive drugs is dangerous while any old physician, without training in psychiatry or psychopharmaceuticals, is fully qualified to administer powerful toxins to the most complex organ one possesses. They can't possibly believe that but it is a measure of how low they are willing to stoop for acceptance. They really should not be allowed beyond the shallow end of the pool.

If you expect sense from the psychiatric community, you are destined for disappointment. They give up eighty percent of their patients without complaint. They labor in the second-lowest paid specialty and throw darts at psychologists.

As the medical industry is now guided almost exclusively by the demands of money, intentionally choosing such a low-paid specialty may provide us with an insight into them that is less than flattering. Their need for acceptance in the medical community must be truly profound.

In describing this little sideshow of a spat between these two parties, it may have come across as being of some consequence. You may have gotten the mistaken impression that training in psychiatry and/or psychology has some value. If I left that impression, I sincerely apologize.

It was brought to my attention that an unusual study was conducted in the late 1970s. I found it a bit surprising that someone had conceived of this particular study. The results of therapy by psychiatrists were compared to the results of therapy by untrained college English professors. There was no significant difference in outcomes.

Many may find that surprising. Personally, I found it amusing. I also found it supportive of the conclusions I have drawn from my research. The logic of that is covered elsewhere.

As cited elsewhere, other studies consistently have shown psychiatrists to be less successful in the treatment of Turbiasis than witch doctors. Why is this so?

The reason is obvious and straightforward. Producing the same results from psychiatrists and English professors tells us that technical training has no effect. All of the vaunted insights, all of the brilliant conceptions upon which their specialty is built is mindless, meaningless blather. All of the years they spent on education in this field were a simple waste.

Am I being just a mite too harsh? No. Don't blame the messenger. Studies of this type did not bring me to the above conclusions. The conclusions are inherent in the studies, studies done by their colleagues, their peers.

However pleased with themselves they may be over their mastery of the mysteries of the human psyche, their efforts in the area of Turbiasis have been, at best, worthless and, far too commonly, harmful, even fatal.

Significant numbers of this profession have sold the safety and well-being of their patients for money, for dinners and shows, for golfing trips, et al. Many have sold their name and reputation to the drug companies for money and ego. Almost all have failed to do due diligence. They have failed to question the lies, the absence of logic, the system. One has to wonder if they can tie their own shoes.

Back in the mid-1990s I came across a bulletin board on the Internet for people with depression. A psychiatrist was a regular poster there. He meant well. He imposed reasonable limits, acknowledging that it was not advisable to diagnose and give too specific advice through that medium. He did offer his expertise free of charge. That was nice, generous and well-intended but mostly unhelpful or harmful.

I recall that at one time he listed various symptoms under two columns: typical depression and atypical depression. Eating too much may have been under typical while lack of appetite was under atypical. The list covered such symptoms as sleeping too much or too little, loss of interest in sex or excessive interest. It gave the appearance of a Chinese menu. Pick from column A or column B.

The problem with such simplistic categorizations is that one may experience all of his symptoms in one column or the other sometimes but at other times experience some from one column and others from the other column. If so, does that person have typical depression or atypical depression or is it possible to have both at the same time. What was designed an easy tool for the psychiatrist is meaningless and useless. Good intentions are insufficient, especially when combined with ignorance.

Therapists are more influenced by their training and current thinking in the field than they are by observations of a patient. Most observe patients only at the most superficial level. A professor of psychiatry stated that a typical clinical psychiatrist learned more about the passenger next to him on a flight than he knew about any of his patients.

A study showed the average psychiatric session for Agmina to be 13 and a half minutes, once every two months. This gives the psychiatrist time to ask the patient's name and scan the patient's record (one should be sure they match), determine if the patient is experiencing any side effects and renew the prescription or change the medication. "Sorry, time's up. Come back in two months."

What is wrong with these people? Let me count the ways:

They spend as little time as possible with their patients.

They fail to get to know their patients.

They prescribe dangerous toxins without any real knowledge of what they do.

They presume their degree confers an expertise over a unbelievably disparate range of specialties, from marriage counseling to schizophrenia.

They actually believe a scientific absurdity to be the basis for mental illness.

They are taught to be objective in dealing with a subjective experience. And never the twain shall meet. To acquire any relevancy they must at least be trained to appreciate the subjective.

They establish a distance from the patient. This is the opposite of what is needed.

They maintain the distance with nonsensical medical jargon.

They intentionally attempt to intimidate with the pretense of being some superior, authority figure.

They fail to create a rapport with patients.

They fail.

A Little Help

In their failures, in their hubris, in their incompetence, in their ignorance, in their betrayal of their charges, psychiatrists also have done irreparable damage to their profession. But, try as they may, they haven't quite managed to earn a place next to the dodo bird. As inept as ever, they just can't get the job done. They need some help.

The goal is not necessarily to do away with the whole of psychiatry. The goal is to get them out of the business of treating Turbiasis with their toxins and ignorance. Help is on the way. As unusual as it may sound, the first step will make their billfolds a little fatter.

The plan is to recruit a few hundred Agmina who have been treated with pharmaceuticals by physicians other than psychiatrists. This should not be difficult, as you remember that they write 80% of the prescriptions for all those colorful little psychopharmaceutical pills.

It has already been established that this group of physicians is essentially without any professional training in the subject. It is also established as a scientific certainty that the drugs they are prescribing are harmful.

The next step is to file a handful of malpractice suits. These suits would all be against physicians covered by the same malpractice insurer. At this point an approach is made to the insurer. The situation is explained. The insurer is asked to institute a policy that no coverage will be available to physicians other than psychiatrists for any treatment of Turbiasis.

The better part of valor would be for the insurer to then recognize his own self-interest and advise all policyholders of the new rules. Absent such recognition the fun would begin. An onslaught of individual malpractice suits would be brought.

Either way the result would be no coverage for the treatment of Turbiasis by general practitioners and other specialties. As I said earlier, the initial effect would be to fatten the bank accounts of psychiatrists. While they now write only 20% of these prescriptions, they will then be the only ones permitted to write them.

Numbers alone preclude psychiatrists being able to suddenly begin writing five times as many prescriptions as they presently do. That will greatly diminish the number written. That will substantially reduce the number of pills sold, the number of pills taken. That will be a major victory.

It will be far too large a story for the media to ignore. Reporting that courts have ruled that unqualified people have been harming patients with dangerous drugs will reduce the numbers of people asking for drugs. There will be only 20% as many physicians telling patients they need drugs.

Although less dramatic, if our efforts cause the insurers to alter policy without recourse to the courts, the word will still get around as to the reasons. Either way the goal of reducing the use of these toxins will be realized.

If the legal route is necessary, success will require the courts to officially recognize and rule that the drugs cause harm. All of the health insurance companies then would need to immediately strike these drugs from their formularies. They won't cover drugs the courts have ruled are harmful and not efficacious. Even psychiatrists would not be permitted to prescribe them. Their prescription pads will become useless. Mission accomplished.

If the legal route is not necessary, there still will be some concern on the part of both health insurance companies and malpractice insurers with regard to covering psychiatrists and permitting these drugs to be used by them. The threat of the next step will be there. The next step will be to challenge the coverage of psychiatrists using psychopharmaceuticals as was done with the other specialties.

We will be able to put a number to the lost revenue for al-Pharma. We will be able to count the number of psychiatrists leaving their specialty. We will not be able to quantify the most important consequences. We will not be able to put numbers on the reduction in misery experienced by Agmina and their families.

Some members of the specialty may be upset with us. That is to be expected even though unwarranted. By their greed, their intellectual lassitude, their failure to give the well-being of their patients priority and an extensive litany of violations of trust they have sentenced themselves. We merely are offering to provide the *coup de grâce*.

Chapter 16

~~Don't~~ Try This at Home

Some people change when they see the light, others when they feel the heat.
Caroline Schoeder

He that will not apply new remedies must expect new evils.
Francis Bacon

The world hates change, yet it is the only thing that has brought progress.
Charles F. Kettering

If you've been paying attention, you may have noticed that, based on the science, based on all of the credible information available, based on reason, based on concern for those suffering from Turbiasis, all psychopharmaceuticals should be avoided. All are harmful. None help alleviate or cure the problems we are addressing.

For emphasis, I will quote from Chapter 10.

"At this point we cannot trace each path and list each organ and each chemical or give numeric values to the degrees of normal functioning of the various parts. The possible variations are unknowable at present. How much commonality and/or difference there is between the involved parts and pathways brought into play by different stimuli is mere conjecture today."

Our lack of knowledge should be seen as an absolute discouragement of crude tinkering. Assaulting the brain with knitting needles, alternating current or massive amounts of poison pills is brainless. The only approach for rational people is to reduce the stress, use methods we know will assist the brain to repair itself and look for other ways of so assisting.

So, what are we to do? How do we help the Agmina? We change. We stop doing further damage. We adopt the credo that the medical profession has abandoned: "First, do no harm." I recommend a total elimination of the use of all of these drugs. But slow down. Those on the drugs must be weaned off slowly and deliberately. We don't need to add to their problems by bringing on drug withdrawal.

One concession could perhaps be made to the use of pharmaceuticals. Being in an active psychotic state can cause some brain damage. There is no appetite to cause further damage nor to allow such to occur, if it can be prevented. If what damage may be brought on by an episode can be reduced or avoided by a medication, an attempt is certainly in order.

What might be appropriate is a sedative. It should be one with minimal side effects and of moderate potency, without liability of habituation or addiction. We are speaking here of an immediate, one-shot intervention, not a continuing course of treatment.

So, the patient's system is clean of psychoactive drugs and the patient is not actively psychotic. What do we do? Remember that Agmina are individuals and the variations you must deal with, both in the people and in the expressions of Turbiasis, are too numerous to completely cover. There are, however, some basic, necessary considerations.

Avoid stress when and where feasible. Reduce stress to the extent possible. Learn better ways of dealing with and reacting to stresses that are unavoidable. Here I am speaking of the external stresses. There are other means available to us that can assist the allostatic system in the physiological realm. We have the knowledge of some ways to bolster the system.

Given the individual, his environment, his resources, the types of stress to which he is most vulnerable and the degree to which those stresses are amenable to avoidance or mastery, the possible ways of handling this are far too many to cover here and too nuanced to cover adequately anywhere. The person with the illness and those available to help bear the burden of deciding on and implementing the specifics.

I recall seeing, some years back, a title at a bookstore, *1001 Ways to Reduce Stress*. It could have been 101 ways but it is unlikely that the author exhausted the possibilities in either case. It is also unlikely that all those methods will work for any particular person.

Find an activity. Find something that is both enjoyable and relaxing. Winston Churchill found two activities. Each served a particular need. He took up oil painting and became a fairly competent artist. The other recreation may seem a mite strange. It was bricklaying. His estate, Chartwell, provided ample opportunity to indulge this activity.

Everyone can find an activity suitable to themself. It could be one that stimulates the mind while being a distraction from certain stresses. It could be something that distracts without imposing intellectual effort. One may, as Mr. Churchill, need both.

If you don't think that you have the requisite artistic talent or interest in bricklaying of Mr. Churchill, there are other options. When I lived in an isolated cabin I could go out on to the front porch or into the woods and scream and yell my head off. It released tension. It reduced stress.

One of the easiest methods of reducing stress is breathing, slowly and deeply. It's easy to begin, continue for a few minutes and stop when distracted. So, just start again until you are again distracted. There isn't any special routine. Just do it frequently during each day.

Even easier than deep breathing is sleeping. Those with Turbiasis often have problems sleeping. Get seven or eight hours nightly, anyway. Your body needs it. Your brain needs it. You need it.

Getting by on three to four hours of sleep, as my manic-depression has led me to do, does not mean that is all you need. Such behavior keeps the allostatic system running overtime. There is insufficient time for the damage to the body and brain to be repaired.

The experiences of my early years put crying pretty far down on my to-do list but for many it is a wonderful release. I would probably be in much better shape if I could more readily cry.

There are a multitude of methods that work. You can find several that work for you. Don't be concerned with what others may think; use what works for you. It's your problem and you can cry if you want to.

This is going to be a bit more time-consuming than writing a prescription. The upside is that you are far more apt to see success. Two requirements here: work at it; and think. Turbiasis rarely cures itself. We must actively pursue our goal and use our brains.

Surely that's not all I have to offer as therapeutic possibilities. True. Not by a longshot. I will briefly cover a few means of improving the odds now and delve more deeply into others further along. I expect that my list is incomplete. The absence of some method you consider potentially helpful perhaps only means that I failed to include it, or think of it. The reason for brevity in some areas should not be construed as my minimizing their importance. It is merely that much better resources are available from others, far more qualified in those spheres.

Eat Up

One of those is diet. Diet can play an important role in this arena as it does in health generally. To make the components the brain and body need to function properly, you must first get them in there.

Tryptophan is the precursor of serotonin. A major source of this is turkey. I am certainly not suggesting anyone eat turkey for three meals a day.

If you can remember far enough back, I don't buy into the common myth that serotonin plays some critical role in depression but, given all the other roles it plays, it's probably a good idea to have some of it somewhere inside of you.

Due to the tryptophan, eating lots of turkey will tend to make you drowsy and serotonin does play a role in the sleep function but it, or some postulated deficiency, doesn't appear capable by itself of being as disruptive in that realm as the sleep anomalies we commonly see in Turbiasis.

Earlier I discussed cholesterol and its part in making cortisol. It can hardly be over-stressed that diet is important in many ways. There have been some interesting studies, primarily in Europe and Korea, that associate low cholesterol levels in people experiencing major depression with violence and suicide.

A Korean study estimated the tipping point to be a level in the neighborhood of 160. None of the reports I have specify whether the low levels were natural or the result of medications. That could be a consideration.

Remembering that cholesterol is metabolized into cortisol, one might think that high levels of cholesterol and the damage cortisol can wreak would be more likely to be associated with violence and suicide.

Cortisol has numerous jobs. It could be that a person's serum cholesterol level is low because another process is using it in a way that has the effect of promoting violence or suicide.

There are other possibilities but that is certainly one that should have been explored. The new model allows for various possibilities to be explored. A simple imbalance of serotonin offers no potential answers.

Institutions seem committed to poor diets. There are reasons for this. They seem to think that, whatever their ostensible mission, their first priority is to save a buck. This appears to them to be an easy and straightforward budget item to target. Just load up on the starches. Starches are generally less expensive than many alternatives. Many books on nutrition barely touch on the perils of a diet heavily laden with starches because they are so well-known and well-accepted.

Some institutions, particularly prisons and psychiatric facilities, have an additional reason for favoring starch. The diets result in lethargy. So? That may be good for the keepers but no one else, especially not Agmina.

There is a great need in Agmina for the entire spectrum of nutrients. There is also a great need for their systems to be energized, not lethargic. The general repair work of the body and brain that is required and the absolutely vital process of neurogenesis demand energetic functioning of appropriate systems.

Avoid all fad diets. Many have the imprimatur of a physician. So what? No medical school offers sufficient education in diet to qualify one as an expert. Diets by different physicians frequently contradict one another. Also, some diets developed or hawked by physicians have proven harmful.

Eat moderately. Eat a wide variety of foods. Eliminate my favorites — eliminate all fried foods. Seriously reduce simple carbohydrates; not all carbohydrates. Vegetables are generally high in complex carbohydrates.

The human body has adapted over millions of years to a particular group of foods. These are the things we ingest that the body knows how to handle. Let's call them the natural foods. The body knows what to do with saturated fats. It has no idea of how to deal with those strange molecules called polyunsaturated fats.

Saturated fats are stable. They do not do strange things when heated to high temperatures, when they are used in cooking. But, polyunsaturated fats are seen by the body as unnatural. They are unstable. They are processed with heat. They are the source of free radicals and other problem-causing factors both before and after we use them for cooking.

Our bodies, our cells need fat; but only the proper kinds of fat. Likewise, our bodies need protein. The other little item our bodies need is carbohydrates. This, as with fats, can be a problem. We need the right kinds of carbohydrates.

Eat moderate amounts of carbohydrates. Avoid simple carbohydrates. Fruits and vegetables contain sugar; not as much as a cinnamon roll but sufficient for our needs. Eating a cinnamon roll will cause your blood sugar level to skyrocket. It will activate the release of insulin, quickly dropping your blood sugar level.

Instability of your blood sugar level will do other things. It will call into action parts of your allostatic system. Your body might start using its protein, your muscle tissue for energy, turn the sugar into fat and store it around your waist. We don't want that, now do we?

Eating natural foods means we have to eat real butter, not that wonderful, synthetic, artificially-colored, artificially-flavored concoction that might fool the taste buds of some people but really can't fool Mother Nature, despite that classic commercial.

We can eat real sour cream. We can eat lots of things we are told, by massive food processing conglomerates, are bad for us. Why would they say those things?

Don't get carried away. The key words are moderate and reasonable. You can actually lose weight on such a diet. It won't be a dramatic 50 pounds a week loss but it can be a healthy 2 to 3 pounds a week.

One more caution, don't make significant cuts in portions. This is why most dieters gain back more weight than they lost. This is the why most serial dieters experience the yo-yo effect.

Trying to lose weight by reducing how much you eat sends a message to the allostatic system. It sends the wrong message. It says you are starving. The system reacts to that message. It slows down your metabolism. That is not the message a dieter wants to send. Your body will adapt to the reduced intake and you will eventually start back up the scale.

Following the above guidelines, surprisingly, can help those who need to gain weight. How? When the body is permitted to operate as it has been programmed to do and given the fuel it recognizes, it tries to find its proper weight. What your body thinks is its proper weight may not exactly coincide with the latest fad or cause people to mistake you for an emaciated high fashion model but it will be able to function better than otherwise.

Easy Does It

The food chain continues getting longer. From the farm to the table, the time and amount of processing continue to increase. Nutrients are destroyed and depleted by time and processing. Supplements are absolutely necessary to the common American diet.

Don't get carried away and clean off the vitamin and supplement shelves at Wal-Mart. A good multivitamin will suffice for most of us, although some recent studies are suggestive that the addition of fish oil can play a positive role for the general population and may have a particular benefit in dealing with Turbiasis.

If you smoke, quit. If you don't, take vitamin C. Smoking depletes vitamin C. A couple of 500 milligram tablets a day will help. The time-release type will help more. If you don't smoke, try to get the amount you need from oranges and other foods.

You should get all of the vitamin E you need from a multivitamin tablet. Vitamin E is an antioxidant, which is good but it interferes with several medications and has not been shown to provide the benefits that many had touted it to have. Mega-dosages of this or that vitamin seem always to fail to live up to their hype. Save your money.

The self-styled health food industry almost daily offers a new exotic herb around which they construct a miracle. While Agmina often desperately want something to help with this or that, they have no patent on desperation. Lots of people get sucked in by these minor league snake oil salesmen. Save your money.

Row, Row, Row Your Boat

As with a good diet, we all know exercise is important to everyone to maintain our health. Agmina receive valuable benefits from exercise beyond their general health. As with diet it isn't necessary to go overboard with exercise. Studies centered around the benefits of exercise on depression, diabetes, heart disease and other problems usually involve only limited amounts of moderate exercise. Thirty minutes a day of walking for five days a week has produced dramatic results in most of these studies.

When depressed, people tend to become less active. Exercise is needed at just that time.

Exercise promotes neurogenesis. Strangely, forced exercise was shown to be even more beneficial in rat studies. Rats that were forced to run the wheel twenty minutes a day had better results than rats exercising the same amount of time on their own.

I am not suggesting Agmina be chained to Nautilus machines or treadmills. It was just a curious outcome I thought worth sharing. The reasons for it may some day become clear and lead to something of more practical use.

Exercise increases circulation of prolactin. Prolactin acts to reduce anxiety and stress by repressing levels of stress hormones and HPA activity. Now you have one more reason to put down the remote.

Exercise has other benefits. It increases brain-derived neurotrophic factor, a growth factor that is known to protect neurons and play a significant role in learning. Although the research is there to prove that exercise can increase learning, one may harbor a modest degree of scepticism when considering athletes in colleges and at the professional level.

Just to complicate matters a little, let me remind you of dopamine. People with schizophrenia were said to have excessive amounts of this neurotransmitter. This comes from the origin of the 'chemical imbalance' fable. The answer was to inhibit it.

However, when dopamine is released from the hypothalamus it is not a neurotransmitter; it is a hormone. In this mode it controls the release of prolactin by the pituitary gland.

Remember, dopamine is involved in the functioning of the central motor system. Does your physician know this? Does the drug salesman know this? Does your local drug manufacturer care?

Charming

Music hath charms to soothe the savage breast. It also has the ability to create savage beasts. For our purposes the former is to be preferred. More than using music just to provide a calming effect, certain music can promote neurogenesis and increase one's I.Q.

The connection between math and music has been shown time and again. A significant percentage of those with a talent for one exhibit greater than average ability in the other. That music containing a high degree of mathematical exactitude has been shown to have positive effects on brain development, primarily by increasing dendrites.

The music of Mozart is noted as being the most mathematically precise. It also is credited with having the greatest positive results. It isn't necessary to limit yourself to a repertoire composed solely of the work of Wolfgang Amadeus.

There is a great deal of good music that will suit our needs. You will find the bulk of it in the Classical genre but there is therapeutic music extant in other types. Few of those three-chord masterpieces for fake guitars composed under the influence in the parents' garage exhibit the needed mathematical fundamentals.

You Are Here

Well, if you have persevered this far, you are probably more than ready for the big one. The most important therapy available to us presently is the establishment of rapport, to bond with the one you want to help. It sounds simple but putting it into practice is not always easy or possible.

A recent study by Swiss and American researchers was reported in the British journal *Nature*. They developed a way to test the effects of oxytocin, a neuropeptide, on the degree of trust people exhibited. The results were significant.

Bruce McEwen at the Rockefeller Institute and others have, in the past few years, found oxytocin to be involved in bonding. Trust. Bonding. There is so much overlap in meaning that which one you prefer is more a matter of personal preference than of semantic exactitude. Bonding and/or trust are necessary to establish rapport.

The production of oxytocin is stimulated in the brains of both mother and child during breast-feeding. Men are not excluded, however. Men and women both have it in their systems.

In addition to the bonding effect, or as an associated part of the process, oxytocin is effective at neutralizing cortisol. This makes a great deal of sense. Cortisol plays the major role in the fight or flight response.

But neither fight nor flight are appropriate to the mother of an infant. It would not be advisable to drop the baby and run nor to drop the baby to engage in a fight. Bonding with others in the group means that the mother is more likely to be surrounded by a support group that will offer protection for her and the infant by fighting for them or aiding them in flight.

The bonding aspect of oxytocin is even better than it may seem at first blush. Not only does it help one to bond with another, the act of bonding actually increases the production of oxytocin.

By reducing the level of cortisol we are altering a process that will result in a reduction of stress. Isn't that what we want? Absolutely. We have a way of reducing the factor that is heavily involved in causing the emotional problems. It has the added virtue of reducing the damage to various parts of both the brain and the body. In the process of reducing stress oxytocin also lowers blood pressure and heart rate.

The researchers cited in the *Nature* article expressed a concern that unscrupulous con men, politicians and others might be able to take advantage of people by using it to increase the level of trust. My first thought upon reading of their worries was that al-Pharma would be the initial abusers of that possible potential.

The application method employed in the study was as a nasal spray. Their results provided only a very temporary effect. More persistent methods will surely be developed. I would recommend relying on generating it naturally and carrying a clothespin in your pocket, if you feel yourself to be threatened by al-Pharma, a psychiatrist, a politician, a used car salesman or other types of con men.

Simply putting oxytocin up your nose is not going to be the answer. al-Pharma will probably try to add an SSRI to it in order to have something they can patent but neither is that the answer, at least for patients. If you have forgotten, thumb back to Chapter 8.

No problem of the brain is simple enough to yield to a nasal spray. We have already seen a smidgeon of complexity involving oxytocin. It causes bonding and bonding generates it. Just ramping up the oxytocin is not a cure-all and, given all of our experience with the brain, there are almost assuredly untoward ramifications lying in wait if we embark on a simplistic, monomaniacal track.

Several years ago the World Health Organization, a part of the United Nations, conducted a couple of studies.

They compared the treatment of Turbiasis in developed countries with that of treatment in developing counties. That simply means rich countries versus poor ones, respectively. The outcomes were unexpected. Results in the developing countries were far better than in the rich ones. They tried again, suspecting that different criteria were used in poorer countries. Once again, the results were an embarrassment to the developed countries.

Support Your Local Witch Doctor

Those conducting the study and others searched for explanations. To them it made no sense that the latest and greatest that modern science had to offer was unable to match their poor benighted brethren.

It should have been no surprise. Smaller studies had shown shamans, witch doctors, to be more successful than the best modern psychiatry had to offer.

There is a simple explanation. They treat the problem differently. They treat it rationally. In many traditional societies one does not go to the hospital alone, be it a general hospital or an asylum. You are accompanied by a family member or friend. That person may do bedpan duty, cook your meals or play other roles. The patient stays connected. The presence of a friend or family member usually has a calming effect.

By contrast, we benefit from our scientific approach. With our enlightened, modern therapies, we snatch the patient away from his family and friends. We rip him away from whatever comfortable routine and environment he may have. We lock him up in a prison, though we call it something else. We introduce him to a very stressful, unstable setting. We force toxic potions upon him. We leave him wondering when, or if, he will ever get out.

We strip him of his rights, his dignity, of any control over his person. We impose what researchers call learned helplessness. And then we wonder why an illness caused by stress doesn't respond positively. We might wonder why witch doctors realize better outcomes with fewer relapses than do the high priests of modern psychiatry.

Establishing rapport with someone takes time. At the hourly rates charged by the professionals, insurance companies are not willing to underwrite sufficient time to accomplish significant results. Given the financial realities of providing proper therapy to a person afflicted by Turbiasis, we are forced to rely on free or very inexpensive therapy.

You Need a Friend

Where are we going to get any worthwhile help for free or for pennies on the dollar? The first recourse in many cases will be family and friends. It is not the perfect solution and should not be the sole answer for anyone. It is reasonably priced though.

Experience or observation will tell all of us that rapport is not so common a commodity that there is an overabundance of it in every family. Estrangement from family, partial or total, is prevalent in many families. My own experience and observations lead me to suspect that disaffection is probably a somewhat more common circumstance for Agmina than for most.

The lack of understanding on the part of family members and the personality disorders that are usually present create a distance. Love does not conquer all. That the member of the family with Turbiasis is loved is no guarantee that there are no strains in the relationships.

If there is an estrangement from family, we would naturally think next of friends. The problem for a large number of Agmina is that they have few or no friends. I mentioned earlier that Turbiasis tends to separate one from others, even from oneself. Volunteers will need to play a primary role in the new system that must be developed.

For those with family relationships that do embody rapport, they are fortunate. While they may be fortunate, their situation is still likely to be less than optimum. Owning an automobile and wanting or needing to get to some destination does not mean that one knows how to drive or how to navigate to that location. There is an essential body of knowledge, experience and ability required. Rapport is the necessary foundation for helping someone with Turbiasis but is not alone sufficient.

I had intended my next project to be putting together a training manual for a certification program for professionals. However, the need for guidance by family, friends and volunteers is too great to defer or ignore. A handbook for the interested public needs to be given priority. In the meantime use what you have or can develop. Use rapport, but add as much common sense as you can muster.

Lesson One

Some things should be obvious but are not. If a person with Turbiasis is delusional, it is not your place to argue with them or convince them of your reality. What you see as delusional is, at least for the moment, their reality. Robert Whitaker relates an appropriate incident in his book, *Mad in America.*

The Agmina claimed that a spaceship was coming to pick him up, at a specific time and place. Rather than try to dissuade him of his error, the counselor accompanied him to the designated place at the designated hour. They waited. The spaceship didn't make an appearance in a reasonable time. He acknowledged that they weren't coming that day. In a few days he was free of that delusion.

Arguing with the person to convince him that he is delusional will not work. Almost everyone stiffens their back when their beliefs are challenged. You would. He would. With an Agmina there is an additional risk. The person may see your opposition as proof that you are part of a conspiracy. Arguing will only make the situation worse.

Had the counselor been a mental health professional he would have tried to argue the client out of his belief. That is what they do. Fortunately he was not a certified mental health professional. He was selected by the project, Soteria, for his empathy. That is, he was selected because he was not a mental health professional.

Soteria was a project funded by the National Institute of Mental Health. The results it achieved were better than the results achieved by drug therapy. It lost its funding. In the NIMH, as with the FDA and elsewhere, the power of al-Pharma is greater than the interests and well-being of those with Turbiasis.

This book will not provide all of the how-to that you will need. However, you can help an Agmina by explaining what you have learned from it.

You can help that person to free himself from drugs. It also will be beneficial for him to understand what Turbiasis really is. The unknown is almost always a source of fear or anxiety.

If he has bought into the 'chemical imbalance' model, the new theory will make more sense, provide more hope and offer the opportunity for him to play a role in his own recovery. You can tell him what you have learned from this book, or give him a copy.

As covered earlier, dual diagnosis is a relatively common problem. If it is a case of dual diagnosis *e.g.*, depression and substance abuse, treatment priority should be given to the depression. Treating the substance abuse when there is an underlying problem of Turbiasis is treating a symptom rather than the fundamental problem.

More difficult, but possible for some people in some cases, is to help one deal with their personality disorders. This comes, if at all, after a working rapport is fully established. It is no more appropriate for a frontal assault than the situation I described above concerning the visit from a spaceship.

I am very hesitant to suggest that any untrained person attempt to intervene in this area but expect that there is a limited number of people in the right situation with a native grasp of what is needed. If you do try, remember the cardinal rule: your role is not to show them the way; it is to help them find their way.

There are a multitude of techniques that show, or claim, some potential for being helpful. Biofeedback was popular for stress reduction some time back. Although it has not maintained that popularity, it can be a useful tool, albeit not a miracle maker. If you have a couple of bucks in your pocket, a set of worry beads might be a good investment.

Claims are made for sleep deprivation. It obviously isn't a method of reducing stress. There is no apparent rational theory behind it. I think I'll wait a while before trying or recommending it.

Further down the food chain are herbal nostrums such as St. John's Wort. Believable studies have not shown benefits. There are potential problems with this and many other herbs. They may have direct effects that are unwanted or interfere with various medications or combine with some drugs or other herbs, interacting in dangerous ways.

Yoga has shown its potential to offer significant help. A superficial use of yoga, while helpful, will not exhaust the possibilities. One should be cautious, however, in pursuing it too deeply. I am only suggesting caution, not avoidance. If one does wish to delve beyond the surface of yoga, it is wise to have an experienced guide. The popular image of yoga is limited to that surface. Yoga, to its devotees, is a serious and rigorous discipline. There is far more to it than assuming a few static positions, breathing deeply and making a funny sound.

For those put off by the alien aspect of yoga, there is meditation. Some may prefer prayer, and it can help those so inclined. But a meditative and reflective kind of prayer is called for, not the sort of supplication or entreaty commonly heard in Sunday morning services.

Eye Movement Desensitization and Reprocessing (EMDR) has been used extensively to treat Post Traumatic Stress Disorder over the past fifteen years or so.

I don't pretend to any familiarity with it. A psychologist with whom I am quite familiar, a nephew, is enthusiastic about it. He and others feel it worth exploring for the treatment of depression. Others think it has great potential in the treatment of related problems.

Laughter is said to be the best medicine. Maybe not, but it definitely has its place. Those with a sense of humor need to exercise it. I intend to collaborate with someone with a sense of humor in any subsequent book, although many will say there should not be another.

Laughter does have a positive effect on many maladies, including Turbiasis. Use it liberally.

An Aside

I have developed a new therapy. It is not a drug but does come under the jurisdiction of the FDA. It is a treatment that could be used as an adjunct to other therapies. The only possible negative side effects would be to a small and easily identifiable segment of the population. It is expected to be somewhat more than marginally helpful in the promotion of neurogenesis but it should not be regarded as a major breakthrough in and of itself.

An establishment or organization with an Institutional Review Board must conduct the research. I have met with representatives of two major universities in an attempt to interest them in conducting the research.

One imposed unacceptable conditions. It was my first impression that they wanted to control the potential financial rewards more than they wanted to control the testing. Upon later investigation I learned how extensive their financial ties are to al-Pharma. Whatever their reasons, I found it difficult to generate any enthusiasm for their involvement.

From the other I received the impression that the person with whom I was dealing was not the one who would be running the study and she was not interested in giving that person the project.

Office politics? Whatever. The end result was another situation that didn't inspire confidence.

If anyone positioned to conduct such research is so inclined, please contact me. The financial potential is not on a scale that would interest al-Pharma.

It makes use of existing technology in a novel way. Using existing technology limits the potential profits from any patents. It would only help those who need help. That should limit the strain on my e-mail server's capacity.

Finally

A limited amount of appropriate training for volunteers and professionals is presently available but there is no certification process yet. That may be remedied in the not too distant future but certainly not soon enough.

The proven techniques for helping Agmina are time-consuming. There is no way around that stubborn fact. The money is not going to be there for time-consuming regimens. Medications or other speedy treatments are at least a generation away and my personal opinion is that it is much more distant than that.

The only answer I can conjure is to depend heavily on volunteers. The numbers may be difficult to reach but the numbers for every alternative fail to add up. It is not an ideal solution but we have to deal with the real world.

Even a dependence on volunteers will cost some money. The necessary training and eventual certification process will not be without some costs. We cannot expect volunteers to bear all of the incidental costs they will face.

A small fraction of the savings that might be realized from elimination of the services presently paid for could be used to support a substantial volunteer program. They could be but developing a strategy acceptable to all parties is not likely to be a tea party.

Professionals will not be able to fully implement the needed aspects of this approach due to constraints of time and money. They can, however, modify their methods in ways that go part of the way. Some is better than none.

Physicians need to play a positive role in the treatment of Turbiasis. They need to be more aware of the role stress plays in the majority of their patients. Earlier we saw that stress is the leading factor in a long list of somatic illnesses. Helping all of their patients reduce stress and the effects of stress is the most needed change in primary healthcare today. As noted earlier, they could check the vagal tone of any patients they consider subject to stress. Other tests could and should be a routine part of assessing stress in patients deemed likely to have a problem with stress. These would include checking blood pressure, serum cholesterol, cortisol and glycosylated hemoglobin.

Although far from adequate, there are some resources available to help both Agmina and other patients deal with stress. Physicians need to identify those resources and point their patients towards them. Simply eliminating the prescription pad as an element of treatment for Turbiasis would do wonders. Medical societies on the local, state or national levels could make pamphlets available to patients that would briefly explain the basics of what it is and how to approach the problem. I am more than ready to assist in any such effort.

As pessimistic as we probably should be about any effort comparable to the need emerging easily or soon, there is sufficient reason for some optimism. We now have a rational model that leads to workable therapies. It is not a panacea. It offers no miracles but it does provide hope to many. It makes it possible to direct resources in ways that will benefit those who need the benefit: Agmina.

Have I found a cure for Turbiasis? Yes and no. There are some who will find themselves free of symptoms by following the thrust of the measures suggested above. Some will not. The methods I cover above are all part of an arsenal for treating Turbiasis. Not all of these will be appropriate in every case. No single method should be considered as the answer.

For such a complex of problems we will need multifaceted approaches. Use everything that works in a particular case.

A native problem of structure, the damage already caused by stress, too great a predisposition to harm from stress or being too greatly damaged by medication can preclude freedom from symptoms. The situation and conditions of the individuals will be the primary factors in determining to what extent these measures prove useful.

Reduction of stress will help. Establishing rapport with others will help. Eliminating all psychopharmaceuticals will help. How much? No one knows. Each person is different and the science is not to the stage of being able to delineate the necessary details of each person's problems. I can offer no guarantees of a complete cure or remission. I can say with complete assurance that many, probably a very substantial majority, will experience significant benefits from following this path.

Finding various ways of reducing stress and developing strong relationships with friends and family need not be confined to those with Turbiasis. As it may strike anyone, it might be advisable for everyone to take those steps. It could even make the Earth a little nicer place.

Having experienced Turbiasis myself, I wish it were possible to completely eliminate it for everyone. That prospect may or may not lie in our future but the path delineated herein is a step in a positive direction. Chemical imbalance is a dead end; for many quite literally.

Appendix 1

Who?

I hope the following list of Agmina will be an inspiration to others. This covers only the 20th Century. It is not an 'outing' of anyone. The names herein were obtained from public sources. It is not expected to be exhaustive but everyone should be able to find someone they admire.

Marvin Aday (Meat Loaf), comic
Alvin Ailey, dancer, choreographer
Buzz Aldrin, astronaut
Louie Anderson, comic
Oksana Baiul, ice skater
Rona Barrett, reporter
Ned Beatty, actor
Samuel Becket, author
Menachem Begin, P.M. - Israel
Danny Bonaduce, actor
Kjell Bondevik, P.M. - Norway
Clara Bow, actor
Cheyenne Brando, actor
Marlon Brando, actor
Art Buchwald, author
Delta Burke, actor
Tim Burton, film director
Barbara Bush, wife of president
Truman Capote, author
Drew Carey, comic
Jim Carey, comic
Mariah Carey, musician
Dick Cavett, writer, humorist
Ray Charles, musician
Paddy Chayefsky, author
Lawton Chiles, governor
Winston Churchill
Dick Clark, TV personality
John Cleese, comic, actor, author
Samuel Clemons (Mark Twain)
Rosemary Clooney, musician
Kurt Cobain, musician
Ty Cobb, baseball player
Judy Collins, musician
Pat Conroy, author
Calvin Coolidge, president
Francis Ford Coppola, director
John Daly, golfer
Bill Dana, comic
Rodney Dangerfield, comic
Sandra Dee, actor
Ellen DeGeneres, comic
John Denver, musician
Tony Dow, actor
Robert Downey, Jr., actor
Kitty Dukakis, wife of Michael

Patty Duke, actor
Thomas Eagleton, politician
Queen Elizabeth of England
Robert Evans, film producer
James Farmer, activist
Philo Farnsworth, inventor of TV
Jules Feiffer, cartoonist
Carrie Fisher, actor, writer
Eddie Fisher, musician
Larry Flynt, publisher
Harrison Ford, actor
Connie Francis, actor, musician
John Kenneth Galbraith, economist
Judy Garland, actor, musician
James Garner, actor
Stan Getz, musician
Kit Gingrich, mother of Newt
Dwight Gooden, baseball player
Tipper Gore, wife of vice-president
Phil Graham, owner, Washington Post
Graham Greene, author
Shecky Greene, comic
Linda Hamilton, actor
Moss Hart, playwright
Mariette Hartley, actor
Lillian Hellman, author
Ernest Hemingway, author
Margaux Hemingway, actor
Audrey Hepburn, actor
Herman Hesse, author
Abbie Hoffman, author, activist
Anthony Hopkins, actor
Janet Jackson, musician
William James, philosopher
Billy Joel, musician
Elton John, musician
Lyndon Johnson, president
Ashley Judd, actor
Franz Kafka, author
Danny Kaye, actor, comic
Margot Kidder, actor
Otto Klemperer, musician
Pat LaFontaine, hockey player
Jessica Lange, actor
Vivien Leigh, actor
Oscar Levant, musician
Joshua Logan, film producer
Jack London, author
Greg Louganis, diver
Courtney Love, musician
Robert Lowell, poet
Camryn Manheim, actor
Dave Matthews, musician
Robert McFarlane, N.S.A.
Rod McKuen, poet, author
Kristy McNichol, actor
Burgess Meredith, actor
Robert Merrill, musician
Kate Millett, author
Carmen Miranda, actor, dancer
Claude Monet, artist
Thelonious Monk, musician
Marilyn Monroe, actor
Alanis Morissette, musician
John Nash, Nobel Prize Winner
Ilie Nastase, tennis player
Stevie Nicks, musician
Vaslov Nijinsky, choreographer
Richard Nixon, president
Deborah Norville, TV host
Sinead O'Connor, musician
Rosie O'Donnell, actor, comic
Eugene O'Neill, author
Phil Ochs, musician
Laurence Olivier, actor
Ozzy Osbourne, musician
Donny Osmond, musician
Dorothy Parker, author
Dolly Parton, musician, actor
George Patton, army general
Jane Pauley, TV host
Charley Pell, football coach
Teddy Pendergrass, musician
Jimmie Piersall, baseball player
Sylvia Plath, author
Jackson Pollock, artist

Cole Porter, composer
Alma Powell, wife of Colin
Charley Pride, musician
Freddie Prinze, comic
Freddie Prinze, Jr., actor
Bonnie Raitt, musician
Mac Rebennack (Dr. John), musician
Jeannie C. Riley, musician
Joan Rivers, comic
Norman Rockwell, artist
Axl Rose, musician
Eleanor Roosevelt, wife of FDR
Kermit Roosevelt, son of Theodore
Theodore Roosevelt, president
Roseanne, comic
Winona Ryder, actor
Yves Saint Laurent, fashion designer
Charles Schulz, cartoonist
Monica Seles, tennis player
David O. Selznick, director, producer
Dmitri Shostakovich, musician
Neil Simon, playwright
Paul Simon, musician
Don Simpson, film producer
Phil Spector, music producer
Diana Spencer, Princess of Wales
Rick Springfield, musician
Rod Steiger, actor
George Stephanopoulos, TV host
Darryl Strawberry, baseball player
August Strindberg, author
William Styron, author
Gordon Sumner (Sting), musician
James Taylor, musician
Gene Tierney, actor
Henri Toulouse-Lautrec, artist
Spencer Tracy, actor
Edward "Ted" Turner, founder of CNN
Jean-Claude Van Damme, actor
Vivian Vance, actor
Kurt Vonnegut, author
Mike Wallace, journalist
Damon Wayans, comic
Tennessee Williams, author
William Carlos Williams, author
Bill Wilson, founder of AA
Brian Wilson, musician
Jonathan Winters, comedian
Tom Wolfe, author
Ed Wood, film director
Natalie Wood, actor
Virginia Woolf, author
Tammy Wynette, musician
Boris Yeltsin, president - Russia
Faron Young, musician
Robert Young, actor

Appendix 2

Suggested Reading

They Say You're Crazy: How the World's most Powerful Psychiatrists Decide Who's Normal by Paula J. Caplan, Ph.D.
Perseus Publishing 355pp. 1995

Blaming the Brain: The Truth About Drugs and Mental Health by Elliot Valenstein, Ph.D.
Simon & Schuster Adult Publishing Group 292pp. 1998

Mad in America: Bad Science, Bad Medicine, and the Enduring Mistreatment of the Mentally Ill by Robert Whitaker
Perseus Publishing 334pp. 2001

The End of Stress As We Know It
by Bruce McEwen, Ph.D. and Elizabeth Lasley
National Academies Press 285pp. 2002

The Truth About the Drug Companies: How They Deceive Us, and What to Do About It by Marcia Angell, M.D.
Random House 305pp. 2004

Let Them Eat Prozac: The Unhealthy Relationship Between the Pharmaceutical Industry and Depression by David Healy
New York University Press 351pp. 2004

Glossary

Ad hoc - Latin: Improvised for a specific purpose. Impromptu.
Ad hominem - Latin: To the man. Attacking on personal grounds (not with fact or reason).
Agglutinative - To combine or add on.
Agmina - People afflicted with Turbiasis (mental illness).
Akathisia - Extreme internal anxiety. Associated with aggressive violence.
Akinesia - Motionlessness attributable to a temporary paralysis. Extremely blunted emotions.
Alumna - Latin: Former student - Feminine - Singular.
Alumnae - Latin: Former student - Feminine - Plural.
Alumni - Latin: Former student - Masculine or mixed - Plural.
Alumnus - Latin: Former student - Masculine - Singular.
Amalgam - A combination or blend of diverse things.
Ameliorate - Make better.
Amenable - Agreeable.
Aneurism - Hemorrhage.
Anthropomorphized - An object or animal having human characteristics imposed on it.
Anti-emetic - A drug that reduces or eliminates vomiting and nausea.
Arrhythmia - An abnormal rate of muscle contractions in the heart.
Aver - To declare or affirm solemnly and formally as true.
Avocation - Hobby.

Axon - Long fiber that conducts away from the cell body of a neuron.
Benign - Harmless, kind.
Bi-polar - An attempt at a cute term for manic-depression but not wholly accurate.
Billion dollars - A considerable sum to you and me but not to pharmaceutical companies.
Blandishments - Gifts or flattery used in an effort to urge someone to do something.
Caveat lector - Latin: Let the speaker beware.
Cipher - Many meanings but used here to mean a nobody or a nonentity.
Commensurate - Equal. Matching.
Conflated - Combined or joined.
Consonant - In agreement with.
Construct - A theory. An intellectual model. A paradigm.
Coup de grâce - French: A deathblow delivered to end the misery of a mortally wounded victim.
Dearth - Shortage.
Dendrites - Short fiber that conducts toward the cell body of a neuron.
Differentiation - Separating similar items based on differences.
Digressive - Irrelevant. Extraneous.
Diogenes - The original Cynic who wandered Greece with a lantern looking for an honest man.
Disingenuous - Hypocritical. Insincere.
Disparate - Markedly different.
Down's Syndrome - Popularly called mental retardation.
DSM - Diagnostic and Statistical Manual for Mental Disorders. Currently in the fourth edition.
Efficacious - Effective.
Imprimatur - Formal approval and endorsement.
Endogenous - Derived or originating internally.
Enmity - Anger. Hostility.
Ensconced - Settled in.

Epicanthic fold - A vertical fold of skin over the nasal canthus giving the eyes a slanted look.

Epiphany - A divine manifestation. A sudden dramatic understanding.

Etiology - The cause of a disease.

Explication - Clarification. Explanation.

Extrapolate - Estimate. Draw information from the specific for the more general.

Factotum - Servant. Underling.

Faux pas - French: A socially awkward or tactless act.

Feral - Wild. Undomesticated.

Formulary - An insurance company's list of drugs for which they will pay.

Harangue - Rant. Loud oratory expressed with strong emotion.

Hubris - Unwarranted self-esteem. Arrogance.

Ideation - The process of forming and relating ideas.

Ideogram - Symbol used to express a concept, a word, as in Chinese, as opposed to an alphabet.

Imperative - Requiring attention or action.

Imputed - Attributed.

Incongruent - Inappropriate. Not corresponding in character or kind.

Intrinsically - In and of itself. Inherent.

Inure - Harden.

Kafkaesque - Surreal distortion and a sense of impending danger. From author Franz Kafka.

Lassitude - Diminished energy. Lethargy.

Luddite - After British labor leader Ned Ludd. One who opposes technological change.

Malfeasance - Wrongful conduct by a public official.

Mea culpa - Latin: My bad. An acknowledgment of one's error or guilt.

Milieu - One's environment.

Miracle - Whatever is the latest drug, device or treatment being touted.

Miscegenation - Marriage between different races.
Misfeasance - Doing a proper act in a wrongful or injurious manner.
Modicum - A small or token amount.
Mollified - Appeased. Placated.
Nonfeasance - Failure to perform a required act.
Nostrum - Old-time patent medicine claimed to cure everything.
Obfuscate - To make unclear. Commonly with intent to impress or deceive.
Orifices - Openings.
Ostensible - Apparently true, but not necessarily so.
Palliative - An agent that removes pain.
Palpable - Tangible. Real. Actual.
Paradigm - Model. Prototype.
Pedantry - An ostentatious and inappropriate display of learning.
Pedigreed - Relates to ancestry, bloodline. I used it as a play on words for having proper papers.
Pejorative - Derogative. Disparaging.
Penchant - Leaning. Preference.
Phlegmatic - Showing little emotion. Chilly.
Phrenology - The study of the shape, size and bumps of the skull as determining character.
Plethora - An abundance.
Post facto - Latin: After the fact.
Precipitous - Abrupt.
Prescient - Knowing beforehand.
Prognosis - Forecast. Prospect.
Protocols - Rules. The design of a research project.
Putative - Supposed. Presumed. Purported.
Raison d'etre - French: Reason for being. The purpose that justifies a thing's existence.
Rapacity - insatiable desire for wealth.
Rapport - A relationship of compatibility and trust.
Rubric - Category.

Rube Goldberg - Early 20th Century cartoonist who drew elaborate, complex and comical devices for accomplishing very simple tasks.
Salient - Prominent.
Sentient - Feeling. Aware. Sensitive.
Somatic - relating to the body, especially as distinct from the mind.
Spurious - Commonly intended to deceive.
Stent - A device for holding open a clogged artery.
Stigma - A symbol of disgrace, shame or infamy. A stereotype.
Syngman Rhee - U.S. client dictator of South Korea 1948-1960.
Synapses - Axon-to-dendrite junction.
Tabula rasa - Latin: A young mind not yet affected by experience (according to John Locke).
Thrall - Bondage. Slavery.
Transliteration - Changing a word from one language to another. Names are done by sound rather than by meaning.
Transmute - Change from one state into another.
Trepidation - A feeling of alarm or dread.
Troika - Triad. Three. From the Russian for a three-horse team used to pull a sleigh.
Turbiasis - Mental illness.
Turgid - Pretentiously lofty in style. Muddy. Unclear.
Tyro - Novice. Beginner.
Ubiquitous - Being everywhere at once.
Vacuity - Inanity. Mindlessness.
Verboten - German: Forbidden.
Visage - Countenance. The human face.
Voila - French: There you are. Literally, see there.
Weltanschauung - German: One's world view.